FAST FACTS FOR
STROKE CARE NURSING

Kathy J. Morrison, MSN, RN, CNRN, SCRN, is a certified neuroscience nurse, a certified stroke nurse, and recipient of the prestigious Pennsylvania State Nightingale Award for Clinical Nursing. As the stroke program manager for the Pennsylvania State Hershey Medical Center, she oversees all aspects of stroke care from prehospital through stroke clinic follow-up. Kathy played a pivotal role in Pennsylvania State Hershey Medical Center attaining The Joint Commission Comprehensive Stroke Center certification and has mentored many stroke program coordinators through the process of attaining Primary Stroke Center certification. Ms. Morrison serves on The Joint Commission Expert Panel for Comprehensive Stroke Center Certification standards.

Ms. Morrison's published works have appeared in nursing journals and neuroscience course curricula. In addition to speaking nationally on stroke-related topics, she is active in community stroke screenings and awareness lectures, and facilitates a regional stroke survivor support group. She established the Stroke Coordinators of Pennsylvania in 2010. She is a member of the American Heart Association Stroke Council and a board member of the Susquehanna Valley American Association of Neuroscience Nurses.

Fast Facts for the NEW NURSE PRACTITIONER: *What You Really Need to Know in a Nutshell,* Aktan

Fast Facts for the ER NURSE: *Emergency Room Orientation in a Nutshell, 2e,* Buettner

Fast Facts for the ANTEPARTUM AND POSTPARTUM NURSE: *A Nursing Orientation and Care Guide in a Nutshell,* Davidson

Fast Facts for the NEONATAL NURSE: *A Nursing Orientation and Care Guide in a Nutshell,* Davidson

Fast Facts About PRESSURE ULCER CARE FOR NURSES: *How to Prevent, Detect, and Resolve Them in a Nutshell,* Dziedzic

Fast Facts for the GERONTOLOGY NURSE: *A Nursing Care Guide in a Nutshell,* Eliopoulos

Fast Facts for the CLINICAL NURSE MANAGER: *Managing a Changing Workplace in a Nutshell,* Fry

Fast Facts for EVIDENCE-BASED PRACTICE: *Implementing EBP in a Nutshell,* Godshall

Fast Facts About NURSING AND THE LAW: *Law for Nurses in a Nutshell,* Grant, Ballard

Fast Facts for the L&D NURSE: *Labor & Delivery Orientation in a Nutshell,* Groll

Fast Facts for the RADIOLOGY NURSE: *An Orientation and Nursing Care Guide in a Nutshell,* Grossman

Fast Facts on ADOLESCENT HEALTH FOR NURSING AND HEALTH PROFESSIONALS: *A Care Guide in a Nutshell,* Herrman

Fast Facts for the FAITH COMMUNITY NURSE: *Implementing FCN/Parish Nursing in a Nutshell,* Hickman

Fast Facts for the CARDIAC SURGERY NURSE: *Everything You Need to Know in a Nutshell,* Hodge

Fast Facts for the CLINICAL NURSING INSTRUCTOR: *Clinical Teaching in a Nutshell, 2e,* Kan, Stabler-Haas

Fast Facts for the WOUND CARE NURSE: *Practical Wound Management in a Nutshell,* Kifer

Fast Facts About EKGs FOR NURSES: *The Rules of Identifying EKGs in a Nutshell,* Landrum

Fast Facts for the CRITICAL CARE NURSE: *Critical Care Nursing in a Nutshell,* Landrum

Fast Facts for the TRAVEL NURSE: *Travel Nursing in a Nutshell,* Landrum

Fast Facts for the SCHOOL NURSE: *School Nursing in a Nutshell,* Loschiavo

Fast Facts About CURRICULUM DEVELOPMENT IN NURSING: *How to Develop & Evaluate Educational Programs in a Nutshell,* McCoy, Anema

Fast Facts for DEMENTIA CARE: *What Nurses Need to Know in a Nutshell,* Miller

Fast Facts for HEALTH PROMOTION IN NURSING: *Promoting Wellness in a Nutshell,* Miller

Fast Facts for STROKE CARE NURSING: *An Expert Guide in a Nutshell,* Morrison

Fast Facts for the MEDICAL OFFICE NURSE: *What You Really Need to Know in a Nutshell,* Richmeier

Fast Facts About the GYNECOLOGICAL EXAM FOR NURSE PRACTITIONERS: *Conducting the GYN Exam in a Nutshell,* Secor, Fantasia

Fast Facts for the STUDENT NURSE: *Nursing Student Success in a Nutshell,* Stabler-Haas

Fast Facts for CAREER SUCCESS IN NURSING: *Making the Most of Mentoring in a Nutshell,* Vance

Fast Facts for DEVELOPING A NURSING ACADEMIC PORTFOLIO: *What You Really Need to Know in a Nutshell,* Wittmann-Price

Fast Facts for the CLASSROOM NURSING INSTRUCTOR: *Classroom Teaching in a Nutshell,* Yoder-Wise, Kowalski

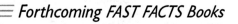 *Forthcoming FAST FACTS Books*

Fast Facts for the MEDICAL–SURGICAL NURSE: *Clinical Orientation in a Nutshell,* Ciocco

Fast Facts for the OPERATING ROOM NURSE: *An Orientation and Care Guide in a Nutshell,* Criscitelli

Fast Facts for the LONG-TERM CARE NURSE: *A Guide for Nurses in Nursing Homes and Assisted Living Settings,* Eliopoulos

Fast Facts for the ONCOLOGY NURSE: *Oncology Nursing Orientation in a Nutshell,* Lucas

Fast Facts for the TRIAGE NURSE: *An Orientation and Care Guide in a Nutshell,* Montejano, Grossman

Fast Facts for the PEDIATRIC NURSE: *An Orientation Guide in a Nutshell,* Rupert, Young

Visit www.springerpub.com to order.

FAST FACTS FOR STROKE CARE NURSING

An Expert Guide in a Nutshell

Kathy J. Morrison, MSN, RN, CNRN, SCRN

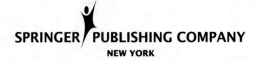

SPRINGER PUBLISHING COMPANY
NEW YORK

Springer Publishing Company, LLC
11 West 42nd Street
New York, NY 10036
www.springerpub.com

Acquisitions Editor: Elizabeth Nieginski
Composition: S4Carlisle Publishing Services

ISBN: 978-0-8261-2717-4
E-book ISBN: 978-0-8261-2718-1

14 15 16 17 18 / 5 4 3 2

The author and the publisher of this Work have made every effort to use sources believed to be reliable to provide information that is accurate and compatible with the standards generally accepted at the time of publication. Because medical science is continually advancing, our knowledge base continues to expand. Therefore, as new information becomes available, changes in procedures become necessary. We recommend that the reader always consult current research and specific institutional policies before performing any clinical procedure. The author and publisher shall not be liable for any special, consequential, or exemplary damages resulting, in whole or in part, from the readers' use of, or reliance on, the information contained in this book. The publisher has no responsibility for the persistence or accuracy of URLs for external or third-party Internet websites referred to in this publication and does not guarantee that any content on such websites is, or will remain, accurate or appropriate.

Library of Congress Cataloging-in-Publication Data

Morrison, Kathy (Nurse), author.
  Fast facts for stroke care nursing : an expert guide in a nutshell / Kathy Morrison.
    p. ; cm.—(Fast facts)
  Includes bibliographical references and index.
  ISBN-13: 978-0-8261-2717-4
  ISBN-10: 0-8261-2717-7
  ISBN-13: 978-0-8261-2718-1 (e-book)
  I. Title. II. Series: Fast facts (Springer Publishing Company)
  [DNLM: 1. Stroke—nursing. 2. Evidence-Based Nursing. 3. Rehabilitation Nursing. WY 160.5]
  RC388.5
  616.8'10231—dc23

2014001221

Printed in the United States of America by Gasch Printing.

*I dedicate this book to my husband, John, for his loving
support, encouragement, and endless patience.*
                                        —Kathy J. Morrison

*Much love and gratitude to my entire family for always
supporting me and my endeavors.*
                                        —Susan J. Pazuchanics

Contents

Part III: Mechanical Interventions for Secondary Prevention

Part IV: Key Elements of Stroke Care

Part V: Post–Acute Care Essentials

Part VI: Primary Prevention Essentials

Part VII: Evidence-Based Practice

Contributor

Susan J. Pazuchanics, MSN, RN, CCRN, RN-BC
Clinical Nurse Educator
Neuroscience Critical Care Unit
Pennsylvania State Hershey Medical Center
Hershey, Pennsylvania

Foreword

Stroke is the fourth leading cause of death and leading cause of disability in the United States today. As our aging population increases in number, we can expect to see a corresponding increase in the number of patients presenting in emergency departments with stroke.

We have seen a dramatic improvement in stroke management in the past 2 decades, particularly since the early 2000s, and nurses have been racing to stay abreast of the changes and *their* increasing educational needs, as well as those of their patients. From the recognition of stroke signs in prehospital care, to the guidelines for inpatient care, diagnostics and interventions, and rehabilitation programs, we now have to consider evidence-based practice guidelines and Food and Drug Administration–approved interventions for the clinician, patient, and the family. A quick reference text to guide nurses is a "must-have" as this disease tests our health care delivery system.

Kathy Morrison is a well-known contributor to the stroke community. She has been actively involved in lecturing, publishing, and research related to stroke patient management. Kathy currently is the stroke program manager at Pennsylvania State Hershey Medical Center and holds a position as adjunct faculty at Pennsylvania State School of Nursing. She also serves on the American Heart Association's

Stroke Council and the Expert Panel of The Joint Commission Comprehensive Stroke Center Standards Committee.

Developing a reference book on a topic that has seen such momentum in recent years is challenging because there is so much new information. The information needs to be relevant, but not overburden the reader who is in need of an answer to a pressing question or situation. Kathy has done an excellent job keeping this book appropriate for everyday use.

Fast Facts for Stroke Care Nursing provides a succinct yet comprehensive review of the evolution of stroke patient management. The text starts with a brief overview of the anatomy and physiology of the brain and cerebrovascular system, tying them to types of strokes, assessment, and diagnostic tools. Acute measures and prevention of secondary injury are outlined and lead us to review the potential complications and finally the rehabilitation of stroke, as well as patient/family education. Particularly helpful is the inclusion of the Brain Attack Coalition, The Joint Commission, and Centers for Medicare & Medicaid Services core measures. Each chapter has helpful Fast Facts in a Nutshell that offer the reader a quick reminder.

Nursing plays a pivotal role in recognizing changes in the patient and coordinating care for the patient along with the other team members. There will be many more nurses joining the specialty of stroke patient care and this book will provide invaluable support to them. Thank you for adding to our knowledge, Kathy!

Linda Littlejohns, MSN, RN, FAAN, CNRN
President, Integra Foundation
VP Clinical Development, Integra Neurosurgery

Preface

For the busy nurse who cares for stroke patients and wants to know that she or he is providing the best evidence-based care possible, this book should be a welcome resource. It is designed to be a practical guide, starting with a brief background on the phenomenon of stroke care improvements, moving through acute care to post-acute care, and finishing with practical pointers for using data to drive performance improvement.

For years I have wondered why there were so few concise reference sources for nurses caring for stroke patients. Nurses want to provide the best care possible, but have lacked practical resources to make that possible. With very little neuroscience content in nursing school, too many professional nurses are intimidated by stroke patients. I feel certain that the more nurses understand about the brain, the less intimidated they will be, and the more great nurses will embrace neuroscience nursing. In addition, once nurses understand the rationale for stroke care standards, they will become strong advocates for following the guidelines. When that happens, the world will be a better place—cared for by passionate, smart neuroscience nurses.

Kathy J. Morrison

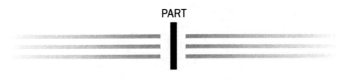

PART

I

Foundations of Stroke Care

Stroke Care Evolution: How We Got Here

Although health care professionals have been caring for stroke patients for hundreds of years, the past 15 years have been marked by dramatic changes in the way care is delivered. Seemingly overnight, stroke care changed from an essentially rehabilitation focus to a true emergency focus. This coincides with the acceptance of evidence-based practice as the cornerstone of the nursing profession. This convergence of nursing professional growth and research-guided evidence has ignited a revolution in stroke care nursing. Although the specialty of neuroscience nursing has been well established for over 40 years, it has shown remarkable growth with the surge of interest in cerebrovascular nursing. Along with advances in neuro-electrophysiology and neuro-oncology, cerebrovascular nursing has contributed to the phenomenon of neuroscience nursing as the new frontier in nursing.

In this chapter, you will learn:

1. The origin of the Primary Stroke Center standards and the certifying organizations
2. The impact of tissue plasminogen activator (tPA) on stroke care
3. The connection between stroke performance measures and stroke core measures
4. Nursing certifications related to stroke care expertise

BRIEF HISTORY OF STROKE CARE

Stroke care nursing is not new. The first time the term *stroke* was noted in English literature to refer to a health condition was in 1689 by William Cole. Hippocrates is credited with coining the word *apoplexy* in 400 B.C.E. to represent episodes of convulsions and paralysis, typically on the opposite side of the body from the injury. He also described episodes of impaired speech, similar to what is known today as aphasia. The ancient Greeks believed that someone suffering a stroke had been struck down by the gods (*Webster's New World Dictionary*, 2008).

Stroke care first appeared in nursing texts in 1890, but with only brief discussions (Nilsen, 2010). The treatment then was supportive care and rehabilitation, but only if the patient survived the stroke and avoided the multitude of secondary injuries that could occur.

The World Health Organization (WHO) defined *stroke* in 1970 as "rapidly developing clinical signs of focal or global disturbance of cerebral function, lasting more than 24 hours or leading to death, with no apparent cause other than that of vascular origin" (p. 2065). This definition is still used today; but with advances in knowledge about the nature, timing, recognition, and imaging of stroke, an update to this definition is needed (Sacco et al., 2013).

Advent of tPA

The year 1996 could be considered the watershed moment for acute stroke care. It is the year the Food and Drug

Administration (FDA) approved intravenous (IV) tPA as the first—and still only—medication for the treatment of acute ischemic stroke. The research outcome was that patients who received IV tPA would have 30% better functional outcomes at 3 months than those who did not receive it. The FDA's approval of IV tPA has become known as the turning point for acute stroke care. Stroke was now an emergency, a "brain attack."

Introduction of the Brain Attack Coalition

The Brain Attack Coalition (BAC) was established in 1991 by a group of neurosurgeons who conceptualized improving stroke care through standardization and evidence-based guidelines. They were inspired by the improved patient outcomes seen with trauma guidelines. The BAC has grown to include membership from 17 professional organizations. This group of highly educated professionals, passionate about stroke care, reviewed over 600 research articles related to stroke care, and in 2000, published Recommendations for the Establishment of Primary Stroke Centers in the *Journal of the American Medical Association*. These recommendations, coming just 4 years after FDA approval of IV tPA, contributed to the buzz that was developing in the more progressive health care organizations around the country; that is, stroke patients should receive care that had been proven through research to improve outcomes. This meant that hospital organizations had the opportunity and responsibility to support evidence-based practice for stroke care.

BAC Member Organizations (Brain Attack Coalition, 2013)

- American Academy of Neurological Surgeons
- American Academy of Neurology
- American Association of Neuroscience Nurses
- American College of Emergency Physicians
- American Society of Neuroradiology
- American Stroke Association
- Centers for Disease Control and Prevention

- Congress of Neurological Surgeons
- National Association of Chronic Disease Directors
- National Association of EMS Physicians
- National Association of State EMS Officials
- National Institute of Neurological Disorders & Stroke
- National Stroke Association
- Neurocritical Care Society
- Society of NeuroInterventional Surgery
- Stroke Belt Consortium
- Veterans Administration

NURSING'S LEADERSHIP ROLE IN STROKE CARE

Despite the unfortunate fact that the BAC did not mention the importance of having nurse coordinators to oversee the immense job of implementing evidence-based standards in acute care hospitals, the majority of organizations came to that conclusion eventually, and a whole new category of neuroscience nurses was born—stroke program coordinators. The BAC made amends for that omission with their 2005 Recommendations for Comprehensive Stroke Centers. In this they detailed the importance of not only educated and competent bedside nurses, but also the importance of having advanced practice nurses (APNs) as well.

Primary Stroke Certification Oversight

Between 2000 and 2004, numerous hospitals reviewed the BAC's Primary Stroke Center (PSC) recommendations and determined for themselves whether all the criteria were met. Many then advertised themselves as PSCs, but who could attest to whether that level of care was actually provided? In 2003, in a study published in the journal *Neurology*, 77% of nearly 1,000 respondents indicated that they met the criteria for PSC, but only 7% actually met all the criteria (Kidwell et al., 2003). It was time for an oversight body for stroke care, similar to the Trauma Systems Foundation. The Joint Commission (TJC) was the first organization to provide PSC certification based on the BAC recommendations, with others following.

Organizations That Provide PSC Certification

The Joint Commission

- Founded in 1951 with the mission of improving health care
- Oldest and largest accrediting and standards-setting organization in health care
- First organization to establish a program for PSC certification in 2003 through its Disease-Specific Care Division
- Certification is valid for 2 years
- www.jointcommission.org/about_us/history.aspx

====*FAST FACTS in a NUTSHELL*

Many nurses have the misconception that TJC is responsible for coming up with the standards for PSCs, probably because they were the first to offer certification, coupled with their reputation as an authority on hospital accreditation. However, it was the BAC that established these standards.

Healthcare Facilities Accreditation Program

- Created in 1945 for the purpose of review of osteopathic hospitals
- Broadened its scope to all hospitals in 1965
- Providing PSC certification since 2008
- Certification is valid for 1 year
- www.hfap.org/about/overview.aspx

Det Norse Veritas

- Founded in Norway and established an American presence in 1897 with the initial focus of risk-management consulting for the maritime industry
- Health care division approved by Centers for Medicare & Medicaid Services (CMS) in 2007 as an accrediting organization
- Certification is valid for 3 years
- www.dnvusa.com/industry/healthcare/index.asp

FAST FACTS in a NUTSHELL

Several states provide stroke center certification either by adopting TJC, Healthcare Facilities Accreditation Program (HFAP), or Det Norse Veritas (DNV) criteria, or through their own distinct processes and criteria. In 2004, Florida, New Jersey, Massachusetts, and New York became the first states to enact legislation or to develop regulations for state-level PSC designation.

CORE MEASURES OR PERFORMANCE MEASURES . . . WHICH CAME FIRST?

Performance measures came first. In November 2004, the BAC, in collaboration with the American Heart Association/ American Stroke Association (AHA/ASA), developed 10 performance measures for DSC Certification for Primary Stroke Centers. These 10 measures were based on evidence from the research of processes that resulted in improved outcomes for stroke patients. Organizations pursuing PSC certification and recertification had to demonstrate compliance with—or performance improvement strategies toward—all 10 of the following measures:

STK-1	Deep Vein Thrombosis (DVT) Prophylaxis
STK-2	Discharged on Antithrombotic Therapy
STK-3	Patients With Atrial Fibrillation/Flutter Receiving Anticoagulation Therapy

(continued)

(*continued*)

STK-4	Thrombolytic Therapy Administered
STK-5	Antithrombotic Therapy by End of Hospital Day 2
STK-6	Discharged on Statin Medication
STK-7	Dysphagia Screening
STK-8	Stroke Education
STK-9	Smoking Cessation/Advice/Counseling
STK-10	Assessed for Rehabilitation

WHY ONLY EIGHT CORE MEASURES?

Core measures have been in place since 2001 as part of the CMS Hospital Quality Initiative aimed at improving the health care delivery process. The original set included only four measures: acute myocardial infarction (AMI), heart failure (HF), pneumonia (PN), and pregnancy and related conditions (PR). In 2008, eight of the 10 stroke performance measures were endorsed by the National Quality Forum (NQF) as core measures and were aligned with the CMS's measures. The two that were not endorsed were dysphagia screening and tobacco-cessation counseling. Dysphagia screening was not endorsed due to the lack of a valid, reliable, standardized screening tool or process supported by research (Alexandrov, 2012), although it is recognized as an important aspect of prevention of aspiration pneumonia. Smoking cessation was not endorsed as it was deemed to have already been met by organizational initiatives and documentation of teaching or counseling provided.

NURSING CERTIFICATIONS

Certifications in nursing signify the attainment of a higher level of knowledge and competence in a specialty area. Unlike licensure requirements, certifications are optional, although the popularity—and number—of nursing certifications continue to grow. As far back as 1997, Barbara Stevens Barnum wrote, "We are in the throes of a love affair with certification in this country, and virtually every RN has a string of (possibly) inexplicable certification initials following their signature" (Barnum, 1997). Certification requirements ensure that continuing education and clinical experience are maintained, a practice proven to raise the level of nursing professional practice. Some of the most popular stroke-related nursing certifications are:

CNRN—Certified Neuroscience Registered Nurse, established in 1978 by the American Board of Neuroscience Nursing (ABNN)

SCRN—Stroke Certified Registered Nurse, established in 2012 by the ABNN

NVRN—Neurovascular Registered Nurse, established in 2007 by the Association of Neurovascular Clinicians

CRRN—Certified Rehabilitation Registered Nurse, established in 1984 by the Association of Rehabilitation Nurses

FAST FACTS in a NUTSHELL

The 1990s were designated as the Decade of the Brain by President George W. Bush in collaboration with the Library of Congress, the National Institute of Neurological Disorders and Stroke, and the National Institute of Mental Health. Numerous programs were developed to bring increased awareness about brain research to the members of Congress and the general public. The 1990s is when acute stroke care got rolling, with the foundation of the BAC, the American Stroke Association, and the National Stroke Association, and approval of IV tPA. Even more has been accomplished since 2000; perhaps the 21st century should be designated as the Century of Stroke Innovation (Figure 1.1).

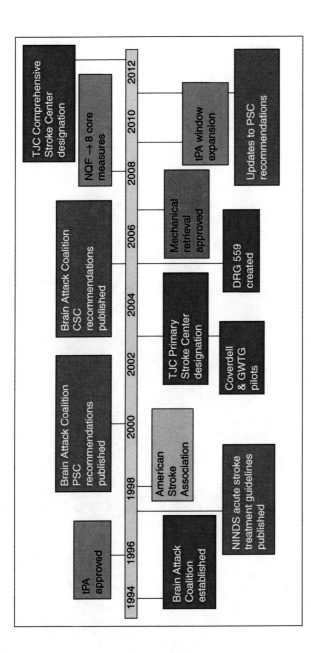

FIGURE 1.1 Acute stroke milestones.

CSC, Comprehensive Stroke Centers; DRG, diagnosis-related group; GWTG, Get With The Guidelines; NINDS, National Institute of Neurological Disorders and Stroke; NQF, National Quality Forum; PSC, Primary Stroke Center; TJC, The Joint Commission; tPA, tissue plasminogen activator.

2

Basic Cerebrovascular Anatomy

Knowledge of the anatomy and physiology of the brain is critical foundational knowledge for neuroscience nurses. Medical science is gaining more insight into the structure and function of the brain, driving the need for nurses to be prepared to care for increasingly complex neurovascular patients. With advances in acute interventions, more patients are surviving large-vessel strokes, requiring expert nursing care. By understanding the function and vascular supply of each region of the brain, neuroscience nurses are able to attribute the symptoms to the area affected, as well as to recognize what is normal versus abnormal presentation.

In this chapter, you will learn:

1. Brain structures and their functions
2. Cerebral vessels that supply these brain structures

BRAIN STRUCTURE AND FUNCTION

The brain is made up of multiple lobes and is divided into two halves, called hemispheres, which are separated by the medial longitudinal fissure (Figure 2.1). The hemispheres

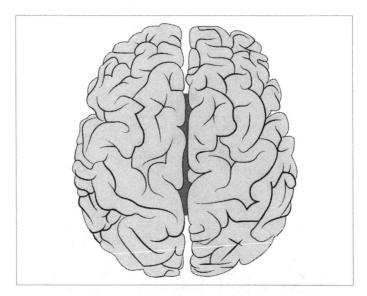

FIGURE 2.1 Brain showing two hemispheres.

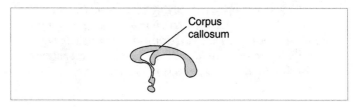

FIGURE 2.2 Corpus callosum.

are connected physically by the corpus callosum, which also facilitates communication between the hemispheres (Figure 2.2).

The outer portion of the hemispheres is the cerebral cortex, also known as the gray matter. It contains numerous sulci and gyri. These folds serve to increase the surface area of the cortex. Beneath the cortex is the white matter, which contains tracts of axons.

The terms *gray matter* and *white matter* originated with early neuroanatomy research using slices of tissue dyed to differentiate structures for microscopic examination. The cells that make up the cortex stained easily, whereas the myelin-covered tracts of subcortical structures did not. Sulci = grooves; gyri = ridges; fissures = deep grooves dividing lobes/regions.

The surfaces of the brain and spinal cord are covered by the meninges, a series of three protective membranes. From outermost layer to innermost layer, the order is:

- Dura mater: Composed of thick, fibrous connective tissue that closely lines the inside of the skull
  - There are two notable dural folds, the falx and the tentorium. The falx separates the right and left hemispheres of the brain and the tentorium separates the cerebrum from the cerebellum.
- Arachnoid mater: A delicate fibrous membrane attached to the dura mater
  - Named for the delicate, spiderweb-like filaments that extend to the pia mater
- Pia mater: A thin membrane that covers the surface of the brain
  - Fits the brain like a latex glove fits the hand, following the surface detail of the sulci and gyri (Figure 2.3)

FAST FACTS in a NUTSHELL

The subarachnoid space is where most major cerebral blood vessels lie. Aneurysms commonly form on these vessels and, when they rupture, result in subarachnoid hemorrhage.

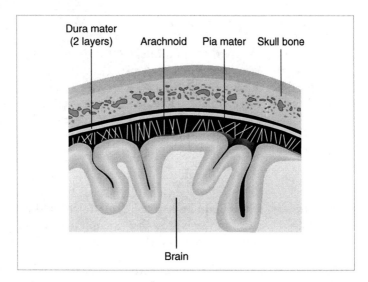

FIGURE 2.3 Meninges layers.

Frontal Lobe

- Anterior/superior portion of the hemispheres
- Functions are reasoning, emotions, judgment, and voluntary movement.
- Broca's area, located in the frontal lobe, is responsible for language production.
- The most anterior portion is called the prefrontal lobe or prefrontal cortex and specifically functions in planning and initiation, personality expression, and moderation of social behaviors.
- The posterior portion of the frontal lobe contains the motor neurons, and is called the primary motor cortex, or motor strip; it is also called the precentral gyrus because it lies in front of the central sulcus, which separates the frontal lobe from the parietal lobe (Figure 2.4).

Parietal Lobe

- Directly behind the frontal lobe
- The anterior portion of the parietal lobe is called the primary sensory cortex, or sensory strip; it is also

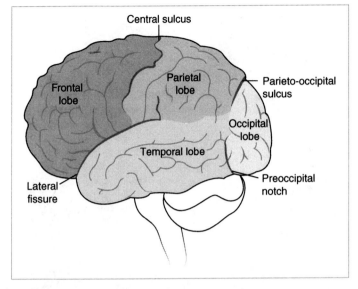

FIGURE 2.4 Side view of brain: frontal, parietal, and occipital lobes and central sulcus and parieto-occipital sulcus.

called the postcentral gyrus. This area functions to process sensory input.
- Right parietal lobe: Responsible for interpretation of the position of the body in accordance to the other objects in its surroundings
- Left parietal lobe: Function includes the ability to understand numbers and manipulation of objects
- Parieto-occipital sulcus: Separates the parietal lobe from the occipital lobe (Figure 2.4)

════════════════════════════ *FAST FACTS in a NUTSHELL*

The homunculus is a diagram that depicts what parts of the body are controlled by the motor and sensory strips. The top of the motor/sensory strip controls the lower portion of the body (legs and feet), whereas the bottom of the motor/sensory strip controls the upper portion of the body (face and arms; Figure 2.5).

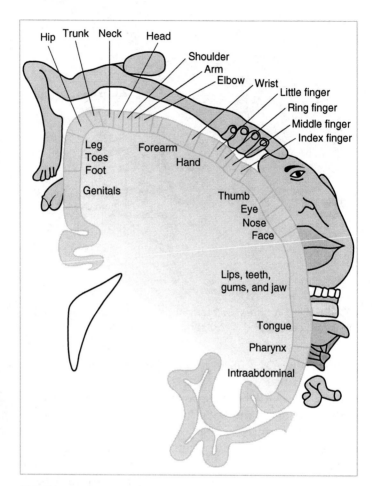

FIGURE 2.5 Homunculus.

Occipital Lobe

- The most posterior portion of the cerebral cortex, and the smallest of the lobes
- Functions are visual spatial processing, color recognition, and motion perception (Figure 2.4)

Temporal Lobe

- Below the parietal lobe and separated from the other lobes by the lateral sulcus, or sylvian fissure
- Functions are hearing, memory, facial and object recognition, and receptive speech
- Wernicke's area is located in the area of the temporal lobe called the primary auditory cortex, and is responsible for hearing and speech processing (Figure 2.4).

DIENCEPHALON: THALAMUS, HYPOTHALAMUS, AND PITUITARY GLAND

- These are located between the hemispheres and are gray matter like the cortical structures (Figure 2.6).

Thalamus

- Serves as a relay station between the cerebral cortex and the brainstem structures
- Relays auditory, somatosensory, visual, and gustatory signals
- Influences arousal and consciousness

Hypothalamus

- Name describes its position; that is, below the thalamus
- Functions in its connection between the cortex and the pituitary gland

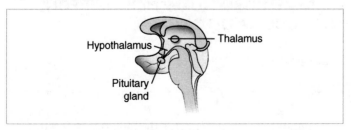

FIGURE 2.6 Thalamus, hypothalamus, and pituitary gland.

- Controls the release of eight major hormones by the pituitary gland
- Controls body temperature, blood pressure, hunger and thirst, sexual behavior, and circadian rhythms

Pituitary Gland

- Located below the hypothalamus, connected by the pituitary stalk
- Referred to as the "master gland" because it directs other organs and endocrine glands, such as the adrenal glands, to suppress or induce hormone production.
- Anterior portion releases hormones that influence blood pressure, metabolism, gluconeogenesis, lactation, ovulation, growth, and immune response.
- Posterior portion releases hormones that influence labor, birth, lactation, and blood pressure.

BASAL GANGLIA

- Subcortical structure, located near the thalamus
- Composed of gray matter and contains the caudate nucleus and the lenticular nucleus, the latter consisting of the putamen and the globus pallidus.
- Serves as the connection between the primary motor cortex and the brainstem, and thus controls voluntary movement and coordination of movement.

BRAINSTEM STRUCTURES: MIDBRAIN, PONS, AND MEDULLA OBLONGATA

Midbrain

- Uppermost portion of the brainstem, superior to the pons (Figure 2.7)
- Motor and sensory tracts pass through the midbrain
- The red nuclei, the substantia nigra, and the origin of cranial nerves III and IV are located here.

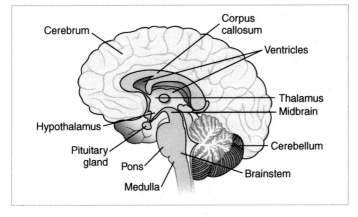

FIGURE 2.7 Midbrain, pons, and medulla.

- Functions to maintain cardiovascular and respiratory homeostasis

Pons

- Located below the midbrain
- Contains motor and sensory tracts
- Serves as a communication and coordination center between the cerebrum and the cerebellum
- Cranial nerves V, VI, VII, and VIII originate here
- Controls sleep, respiratory drive, swallowing, hearing, balance, bladder control, taste, eye movement, facial expression, and sensation
- The reticular formation, which controls consciousness, is located here.

Medulla Oblongata

- Lowest portion of the brainstem, connecting to the spinal cord at the foramen magnum
- Controls respiratory and heart rates, and digestive processes as well as vomiting, coughing, sneezing, swallowing, and balance.
- Cranial nerves IX, X, and XII originate here.

Cerebellum

- Also referred to as the "little brain"
- Located below the cortex and behind the brainstem
- Communicates with the pons and spinal cord to coordinate motor movement and maintain balance
- Contributes to cognitive function, particularly language, in ways that are not yet well understood

BRAIN VASCULATURE

The entire blood supply of the brain depends on two sets of branches from the aorta. The internal carotid arteries are branches of the common carotid arteries, and the vertebral arteries arise from the subclavian arteries (Figure 2.8).

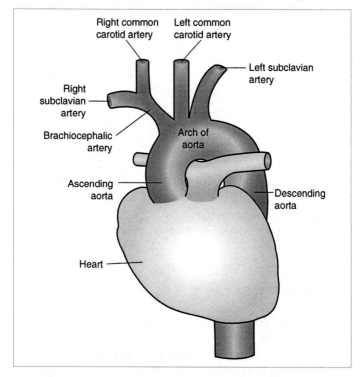

FIGURE 2.8 Aortic arch and subclavian and carotids.

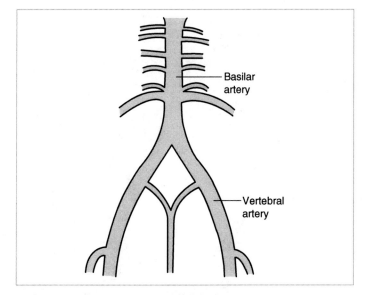

FIGURE 2.9 Vertebral and basilar arteries.

The internal carotid arteries branch to form two major cerebral arteries, the anterior and middle cerebral arteries. The right and left vertebral arteries come together at the level of the pons to form the midline basilar artery (Figure 2.9).

The Circle of Willis

- Internal carotid arteries
- Anterior cerebral arteries
- Anterior communicating artery
- Posterior cerebral arteries
- Posterior communicating arteries
- NOT considered to be part of the circle of Willis (Figure 2.10): the middle cerebral arteries, vertebral arteries, and the basilar artery

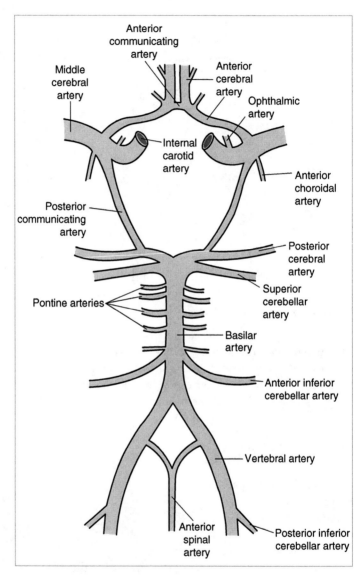

FIGURE 2.10 Circle of Willis.

As much as 50% to 75% of the population has an incomplete circle of Willis, reminding us that collateral circulation is a very important concept in cerebrovascular anatomy. There have been 22 variations of the circle of Willis documented.

Anterior Circulation

- Supplies the anterior portion of the cerebrum—the frontal lobe, temporal lobes, and majority of parietal lobes
- Comprised of the internal carotid arteries, middle cerebral arteries, anterior cerebral arteries, and the anterior communicating artery
- **The internal carotid arteries** (ICA) serve as a connection between the aorta and the anterior brain.
- **The middle cerebral arteries** (MCA) supply blood to most of the frontal and parietal lobes, inferior portion of the temporal lobes, the internal capsule, and the basal ganglia.
- **The anterior cerebral arteries** (ACA) supply blood to the medial portion of the frontal lobe, the medal and superior portions of the parietal lobes, and portions of the corpus callosum, basal ganglia, and internal capsule.
- **The anterior communicating artery**'s only function is as a connection between left and right anterior cerebral arteries.

Posterior Circulation

- Supplies the posterior portion of the cerebrum—the posterior parietal lobes, occipital lobe, cerebellum, and brainstem
- Comprised of the vertebral arteries, basilar artery, posterior cerebral arteries, and the posterior communicating arteries

- **The vertebral arteries** serve as a connection between the subclavian arteries (which arise from the aorta) and the posterior brain.
- **The basilar artery** supplies blood to the cerebellum via the posterior inferior cerebellar arteries, the anterior inferior cerebellar arteries, and the superior cerebellar arteries. It also supplies blood to the pons.
- **The posterior cerebral arteries** (PCA) provide blood to the occipital lobe, inferior portion of the temporal lobe, and the thalamus.
- **The posterior communicating arteries** serve as a connection between anterior and posterior portions of the circle of Willis.

Penetrating Arteries

- Smaller branches of the large cerebral arteries that extend throughout the brain tissue, providing blood flow to all areas of the brain
- Overlap of these vessels accounts for "collateral" flow
  - For instance, if a distal portion of the middle cerebral vessel is occluded, the area it normally supplies can be perfused by a distal branch of nearby vessels. But if a proximal portion of the middle cerebral artery is occluded, there will be a large area of infarction that may not be able to be supplied by smaller, nearby vessels (Alexander, 2013).

CEREBRAL VENOUS CIRCULATION

- Divided into two categories: superficial and deep
- Dural venous sinuses (also called dural sinuses, cerebral sinuses, or cranial sinuses) are venous channels found between layers of dura mater in the brain.
- The venous sinuses collect the blood from the brain and empty into the internal jugular veins. The jugular veins are essentially the only drainage of the brain (Figure 2.11).

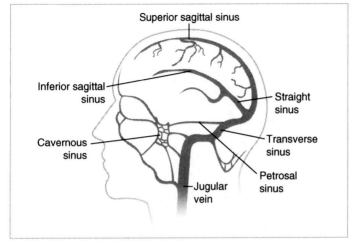

FIGURE 2.11 Venous system, jugular veins.

3

Stroke Types

The brain is a remarkably complex organ, with a vast array of structures and functions. Therefore, a stroke for one person does not necessarily present exactly like the stroke for another person. Coding guidelines may link hemorrhagic and ischemic strokes under the same reimbursement group, but that is where the similarities end. In fact, many neurosurgeons do not refer to subarachnoid hemorrhage as a stroke, and they are reluctant to use the term stroke *for their intracerebral hemorrhage patients as well. These patients are often cared for in the same neuroscience unit, or stroke unit, but the mechanisms of injury are quite different. It is important for neuroscience nurses to understand the unique differences between the types of stroke so that they can understand the differences in care and recovery. Some of the etiologies and risk factors are the same—hypertension, atherosclerosis, and smoking— and we can all agree that regardless of the type, all strokes are vascular catastrophes.*

In this chapter, you will learn:

1. Etiologies of each type of hemorrhagic stroke
2. Distinction among thrombotic, embolic, and lacunar strokes
3. Different types of large vessel strokes
4. Latest definition of transient ischemic attacks (TIAs)

FAST FACTS in a NUTSHELL

Patients who present with minimal symptoms, but deteriorate rapidly, are likely to be having hemorrhagic strokes. Conversely, patients who present with significant deficits, and improve quickly, are likely having ischemic strokes or TIAs.

HEMORRHAGIC STROKE

Twenty percent of strokes are hemorrhagic strokes that happen when a blood vessel ruptures in or near the brain, disrupting blood flow to a part of the brain. The two main types of hemorrhagic strokes are subarachnoid hemorrhage (SAH) and intracerebral hemorrhage (ICH).

Subarachnoid Hemorrhage

- Ruptured cerebral aneurysms are the cause of 85% of SAHs. This causes blood to collect in the subarachnoid space, preventing it from getting into the brain tissue (parenchyma) by the pia mater. Referred to as aSAH, the "a" designates that the subarachnoid hemorrhage is caused by an aneurysm.
- Aneurysms are weakened "ballooned" segments of arterial walls. Over time, and in the presence of hypertension, the aneurysm walls become stretched to the point of breaking.
- Due to the pressure of the blood spurting from the aneurysm, the most common symptom is "the worst headache of my life."

- Most common sites for aneurysms are the carotid–posterior communicating artery junction and the anterior cerebral–anterior communicating artery junction.
- Other causes are sepsis, anticoagulation, and trauma.
- Large amounts of subarachnoid blood can block circulation of cerebrospinal fluid (CSF) resulting in hydrocephalus; this usually occurs later during recovery and may appear as progressive dementia. If it occurs early, it is associated with cerebral vasospasm.
- Cerebral vasospasm occurs due to cerebral arteries in the subarachnoid space being surrounded by blood, which is irritating to the muscular arterial walls, resulting in spasms.
- Mortality rate at 30 days is 50%.

Aneurysm Types

Saccular, also known as (a.k.a.) "berry" due to its shape	• Occur at arterial bifurcations and branches of the large arteries at the base of the brain—the circle of Willis • 80%–90% of cerebral aneurysms
Fusiform	• Outpouching of artery that is expanded in all directions • Has no stem and seldom ruptures
Infective, a.k.a. mycotic aneurysm (Note: This is a misnomer as most are from a bacterial source, and the term *mycotic* indicates a fungal source.)	• Infectious emboli mainly originate in left-sided bacterial endocarditis • Mortality rate is 30% for unruptured, 80% for ruptured • Can produce aSAH or ICH depending in which vessel the emboli lodges

Intracerebral Hemorrhage

ICH is also known as intraparenchymal hemorrhage (IPH).

- Caused by rupture of a penetrating artery, which releases blood directly into the brain tissue; in essence, a hematoma in the brain.
- Hypertension is the single most important risk factor due to dilatation of the cerebral vessels, separating the

normally tight endothelial junctions of the blood–brain barrier, thus lowering the threshold for intracerebral hemorrhage.

- Fifty percent of hypertensive ICHs occurs in the basal ganglia (rupture of lenticulostriate branches of the middle cerebral artery [MCA]), whereas 33% occur in the cerebral hemispheres (rupture of penetrating cortical branches of the anterior, middle, and posterior cerebral arteries).
- Other risk factors are anticoagulation, cigarette smoking, alcohol consumption (more than two drinks daily), cocaine or amphetamine use, malignant neoplasms, and arteriovenous malformations (AVMs).
- AVMs are abnormal vascular beds in which blood flows directly from arteries (with muscular walls) into veins (walls without muscles). The result is weakening and eventual rupture of the venous wall causing ICH.
  - AVMs vary in size and can be found anywhere in the nervous system.
  - Unruptured AVMs cause few physical symptoms, thus they are often undetected.
- Mortality rate at 30 days is 34% to 50%; the mortality rate is much higher for those who are comatose on arrival.
- Incidence is about twice as frequent as SAH.

Intraventricular Hemorrhage

- Blood in the ventricles is usually secondary to SAH or ICH.
- Primary intraventricular hemorrhage (IVH) is most common with traumatic brain injury.
- Once blood is in the ventricles, it can occlude the arachnoid villi that drain the CSF into the venous system, similar to the effect of subarachnoid blood. If this occurs, CSF builds up in the ventricular system and hydrocephalus develops.

> *Parenchyma* means brain tissue. IPH and ICH are often used interchangeably to mean bleeding within the brain tissue.

ISCHEMIC STROKE

Eighty percent of all strokes are ischemic strokes that occur due to lack of blood to part of the brain caused by narrowing or occlusion of vessels or by systemic hypotension. High blood pressure is the most common risk factor because it damages the intima of blood vessels and causes hypertrophic cardiomyopathy, which leads to atrial fibrillation. Other risk factors are cigarette smoking, uncontrolled diabetes, high cholesterol, physical inactivity and obesity, and certain blood disorders. Systemic hypoperfusion is a little-understood cause of stroke; it occurs when the systemic blood pressure is too low and too little blood reaches the brain.

THROMBOTIC STROKE

- Caused by a stationary blood clot (thrombus) or stenosis in an artery going to the brain.
- Blood clots usually form in arteries damaged by plaque.
- Plaque accumulation occurs over time, resulting in narrowing (stenosis) of the vessel lumen.

EMBOLIC STROKE

- Caused by a traveling clot (embolus) that is formed elsewhere (usually in the heart or neck arteries).

LACUNAR STROKE

- Caused by occlusion of smaller, penetrating arteries, blocking blood flow to small portions of the brain
- Also referred to as "pure motor" or "pure sensory" stroke because the territory of infarct is so small as to only affect motor or sensory fibers, usually not both. The surrounding brain tissue often quickly takes over the function of the infarcted territory, thus the symptoms may only last a few hours.

FAST FACTS in a NUTSHELL

In the past, lacunar strokes were often mistaken for TIAs because the symptoms only lasted a few hours, with no imaged infarct. Improved imaging has made it possible to see tiny infarcts, even in the case of symptom resolution.

WATERSHED STROKE

- Occurs at the junction of distal fields of two nonanastomosing arterial systems
- More common in the presence of vascular disease
- There are two types:
  - Cortical watershed (CWS): Between the territories of the anterior cerebral artery (ACA), MCA, and posterior cerebral artery (PCA)
  - Internal watershed (IWS): In the white matter along and slightly above the lateral ventricle, between the deep and the superficial arterial systems of the MCA, or between the superficial systems of the MCA and ACA
- Caused by systemic hypoperfusion or microemboli from carotid artery disease

SILENT STROKES

- Ischemic: Imaging or pathophysiological evidence of infarction without a history of acute neurologic dysfunction attributable to the lesion
- Hemorrhagic: Focal collection of chronic blood products within the brain parenchyma, subarachnoid space, or ventricular system on neuroimaging or neurophysiological exam that is not caused by trauma and without a history of acute neurologic dysfunction attributable to the lesion (Sacco et al., 2013).

LARGE-VESSEL SYNDROMES

- Occur when the blood supply is suddenly restricted or occluded in one of the large cerebral arteries, resulting in a "syndrome" or specific set of symptoms that are often dramatic
- Must be differentiated from gradual onset of occlusion, which allows for collateral circulation to expand to assume the responsibility of supplying that region with blood supply, and stroke does not necessarily occur
- Symptoms are dependent on the area of the specific artery that is affected: Proximal occlusions will result in a broader set of symptoms, whereas distal occlusions will result in smaller territories of ischemia, thus a smaller set of symptoms.

ACA Syndrome

- Signs and symptoms are contralateral hemiparesis of lower limbs (remember the homunculus in Chapter 2), urinary incontinence, and apraxia.

MCA Syndrome

- Signs and symptoms are contralateral hemiparesis and hemisensory loss in the face and arms.
- If the dominant side is affected, speech impairments occur, particularly aphasia because Broca's and Wernicke's areas are part of the MCA territory.
- If the occlusion is proximal, at the origin of the MCA, the result is a devastating, large territory stroke, with 80% mortality.

Vertebral Artery Syndromes

- Signs and symptoms vary considerably depending on the area affected.
- The most common syndromes are:
  - Wallenberg's syndrome: Nausea, vomiting, and vertigo, nystagmus, tachycardia, dysarthria, dysphagia, imbalance, and crossed signs
  - Cerebellar infarction: Incoordination, ataxia, dysarthria
  - Locked-in syndrome: Caused by infarction of upper central pons; quadriplegia with preserved consciousness
  - PCA occlusion: Hemianopia and macular sparing

FAST FACTS in a NUTSHELL

The MCA is the most common site for ischemic stroke. Because it supplies the face and arm territory of the motor/sensory strip, as well as the speech center territories, it makes sense that the FAST mnemonic (face, arm, speech, time) is so popular—these are the most common signs of stroke.

4

Physiology of Stroke

Understanding the different types of stroke is important in caring for stroke patients. Understanding the
physiology of the specific type of stroke will enhance
the nurse's ability to anticipate complications and
focus assessment accordingly. The initial insult of
a stroke is just the beginning . . . the changes that
occur in the brain during the subsequent hours
and days are what separate the neuroscience nurse
from non-neuroscience colleagues. Ischemic stroke
and hemorrhagic strokes have unique physiologies
with one definite common characteristic—they can
change suddenly and the changes are often subtle
at first.

In this chapter, you will learn:

1. What happens in the ischemic cascade
2. How the penumbra develops
3. The effect of blood when it is *outside* the blood vessels

FAST FACTS in a NUTSHELL

The brain represents only 2% of the body's weight, but it uses about 25% of the body's oxygen supply and 70% of the glucose (Brass, 2002). Unlike muscles, the brain cannot store nutrients, and thus it requires a constant supply of glucose and oxygen. No wonder the first symptom of hunger is often sleepiness or headache.

PHYSIOLOGY OF ISCHEMIA

- Normal cerebral blood flow is 45 to 60 mL/100 g/min. When it drops below 18 mL/100 g/min, brain tissue infarction can occur if cerebral blood flow is unresolved for up to 4 hours. The process is known as the ischemic cascade.
- The ischemic cascade is a series of biochemical reactions that are initiated within minutes of brain ischemia.
  - Carbon dioxide retention and adenosine triphosphate (ATP) breakdown occur, activating sodium/hydrogen exchange transporters.
  - Disruption of normal cellular exchange results in cell death.
  - Cell death releases toxic chemicals that damage the blood–brain barrier.
  - Large molecules, such as albumin, pass through the damaged barrier, pulling water with them by the process of osmosis.
  - The result is tissue swelling and edema—the ischemic penumbra.

ISCHEMIC PENUMBRA

- The ischemic penumbra is the area surrounding the infarcted tissue.

- The area is still viable, often supported by collateral circulation, but is at risk of proceeding to infarction, like the core of the stroke.
- If the area proceeds to infarct, it is referred to as "extending the stroke," since the core has now been enlarged.
- The tissue is swollen, resulting in diminished function, increased intracranial pressure (ICP), and somnolence.
- Resolution of edema generally occurs within 72 hours, demonstrated by improvement of some deficits and by patients being more awake and alert (Figure 4.1).

══════════════════════════════*FAST FACTS in a NUTSHELL*

Understanding the physiology of the penumbra will help the neuroscience nurse to educate the patient's family, and allay some of their anxiety during the first few days. For example, a patient with a right middle cerebral artery (MCA) infarct is admitted with left arm weakness. On day 2, the patient is hard to arouse and now the left leg is not working properly either, due to the penumbra swelling into the motor strip area controlling the leg. The nurse can provide this explanation, along with reassurance of close monitoring and careful medical management, indicating that in another day or two, the swelling will subside, the patient will be more awake, and the leg will work again.

PHYSIOLOGY OF HEMORRHAGIC STROKE

Intracerebral Hemorrhage

- Hypertensive intracerebral hemorrhage (ICH) results in an inflammatory response with accompanying edema very similar to the ischemic penumbra; however, its duration is longer than that of the ischemic penumbra.
- The resulting increase in intracranial pressure (ICP) contributes to a reduction in venous outflow, ischemia

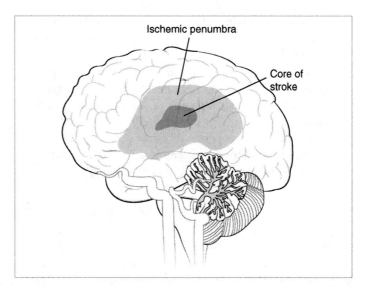

FIGURE 4.1 Ischemic penumbra.

(which initiates the ischemic cascade), and breakdown of the blood–brain barrier.
- Up to 73% of spontaneous ICHs expand over the first 24 hours (Davis et al., 2006)

Subarachnoid Hemorrhage

- Blood is irritating to the exterior surfaces of large cerebral arteries that lie in the subarachnoid space.
- Release of serotonin from the extravasated platelets induces vasospasm that reduces or even stops flow through that artery.
- Secondary ischemic stroke occurs in 30% of these patients, a condition referred to as delayed cerebral ischemia (DCI).
- Cerebral edema also develops due to effects on the blood–brain barrier, contributing to increased ICP.
- Release of catecholamines results in cardiac abnormalities, such as arrhythmias, tachycardia, and hypertension, as well as increased troponin levels.

5

Associated Stroke Disorders

The brain is a complex organ with a complex vascular system. The disorders discussed in this chapter are not viewed as types of stroke, but can lead to stroke. Transient ischemic attack (TIA), in particular, can be a difficult condition to diagnose with confidence.

In this chapter, you will learn:

1. Why carotid dissection can lead to stroke
2. How an arteriovenous fistula is different from an arteriovenous malformation

TRANSIENT ISCHEMIC ATTACK

- Focal neurologic deficits similar to stroke symptoms, but with complete resolution of deficit and no MRI and/ or computed tomography (CT) findings of acute cerebral infarction (Easton et al., 2009)
- Historically, TIA was defined by time-based parameters (i.e., symptom resolution within 24 hours)

- With improved CT and MRI technology, definition is now by tissue-based parameters (i.e., absence of infarction on brain imaging, along with complete resolution of symptoms).

FAST FACTS in a NUTSHELL

TIA is to stroke what angina pectoris is to myocardical infarction (MI) . . . a warning sign. Up to 33% of TIA patients will experience a stroke sometime in the future. Another term for TIA is mini-stroke; some practitioners incorrectly use the term mini-stroke when referring to tiny, lacunar strokes, which has led to considerable confusion.

CEREBRAL VENOUS THROMBOSIS

- Presence of a clot in the dural venous sinuses resulting in blocked drainage from the brain
- Uncommon and frequently unrecognized type of stroke, mostly affecting young people
- Most common causes are hypercoagulable conditions and oral contraceptive use
- 40% of patients present with ICH

DISSECTION—CAROTID AND VERTEBRAL ARTERIES

- Develops when a tear occurs in the intima of the vessel and blood collects between the linings. This not only creates an occlusion, but also provides a source for microemboli to form along the tear.
- Numerous tiny infarcts in a hemisphere are a clue that carotid artery dissection may be present.
- Vertebral artery dissection is much less common.

- Both are more prevalent in young people and in the presence of trauma to the head or neck, but can occur spontaneously (Figure 5.1).

Women at a hair salon, hyperextending their necks at the wash sink, men lifting weights (increases in chest pressure/blood pressure), and chiropractic manipulation have been reported to be related to carotid artery and vertebral artery dissection. However, the majority of dissections are considered "spontaneous" with no known cause.

MOYA MOYA DISEASE

- A rare and progressive disease caused by arterial occlusion in the basal ganglia.
- Name means "puff of smoke" due to the characteristic appearance of a tangle of tiny vessels formed to compensate for the occlusion.
- Primarily occurs in children, presenting as ischemic stroke or TIA

In adults, it presents as intracerebral hemorrhage (ICH) due to recurring clots in the fragile vessels.

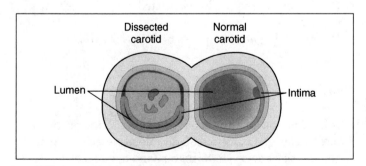

FIGURE 5.1 Carotid dissection. Right diagram represents normal carotid; left diagram represents 100% occlusion.

HYPERCOAGULABLE CONDITIONS

- Clotting disorders in which the blood clots under conditions in which it normally would not
- Most common hypercoagulable conditions are factor V Leiden, protein S and C deficiencies, prothrombin gene mutation, and elevated homocysteine levels.
- The presence of cancer, as well as numerous chemotherapy agents, are known to be prothrombotic as well.

FAST FACTS in a NUTSHELL

It is sad, but not uncommon, for patients who come to the hospital with acute stroke symptoms to also learn that they have cancer. The prothrombotic nature of the cancer creates the potential for clots to form, and, if the clots reach the brain, cause a stroke.

AMYLOID ANGIOPATHY

- Accumulation of abnormal proteins (amyloid) in small cerebral arteries over the surface of the hemispheres
- Progressive arterial narrowing leads to ischemia
- Accumulation also weakens vessels leading to intracerebral hemorrhage.
- Condition is frequently associated with Alzheimer's disease.
- Definitive diagnosis requires brain tissue sample.

VASCULITIS

- Inflammation of the blood vessels that can result in narrowing or occlusion of the blood vessels, and in some cases, aneurysm formation and hemorrhage
- Possible causes are immune system abnormalities, infections, cancer, and rheumatoid arthritis.

ARTERIOVENOUS FISTULA

- Abnormal connection that develops between an artery and a vein, resulting in blood traveling under arterial pressure moving directly into a vein. Vein walls are without muscles, thus are not built for arterial pressure.
- An arteriovenous fistula (AVF) is different from an arteriovenous malformation (AVM) in that AVMs are found within the brain tissue, whereas AVFs develop in the dura or arachnoid maters.

CAVERNOUS ANGIOMA

- A blood vessel abnormality characterized by large, adjacent capillaries with little or no intervening brain. The blood flow through these vessels is slow and the vessels typically hemorrhage in small amounts with bleeding episodes separated by months or years.

6

Stroke Diagnostics

Time is brain, so during an acute stroke workup, diagnostic tests must be prioritized carefully in order to maximize their value without compromising brain tissue viability. Blood glucose, tested via a finger stick by prehospital personnel, is a valuable diagnostic test that can differentiate hypoglycemia-induced symptoms from those produced by cerebral ischemia. Brain imaging is the first line of diagnostics once the patient arrives in the emergency department (ED) in order to clarify the cause of neurologic symptoms. For most organizations, a nonenhanced computed tomographic (NECT) scan is the imaging done emergently to rule out hemorrhage, detect the ischemic tissue, and exclude other possible mimics of stroke (e.g., neoplasm, multiple sclerosis, etc.). An electrocardiogram (EKG) and blood tests are done soon after to provide other critical information to facilitate rapid treatment decisions. An echocardiogram is done during the first 24 to 48 hours of hospitalization, and, depending on the patient's presentation, other diagnostics such as lumbar puncture, transcranial Doppler, chest x-ray, electroencephalogram (EEG), and hypercoagulable lab tests may be performed.

In this chapter, you will learn:

1. The distinctions among CT/CTA/CTP and MRI/DWI/MRA/ MRP/MRV
2. The utility of transthoracic and transesophageal echocardiogram
3. The role of transcranial Doppler (TCD) in stroke care

FAST FACTS in a NUTSHELL

In brain imaging, the term "angio" refers to blood vessels, so a CTA (CT angio) or MRA (MR angio) utilizes contrast agents and visualizes the vasculature. The term "perfusion" refers to the adequacy of the blood supply to the brain tissue.

BRAIN IMAGING

- Computed tomographic (CT) scan
  - First done in 1971; *tomography* is from the Greek word "tomos" meaning "slice" or "section" and "graphia" meaning "describing"
  - CT without contrast (NECT)
    - First-line diagnostic due to its speed and availability in comparison to magnetic resonance imaging (MRI) (Latchaw et al., 2009)
    - Gold standard for detection of intracerebral hemorrhage, and superior to lumbar puncture in detection of subarachnoid hemorrhage
  - CT angio (CTA)
    - Depicts the occlusion site, helps grade collateral blood flow, and helps characterize carotid atherosclerotic disease
    - Requires use of contrast material
  - CT perfusion (CTP)
    - Delineates the ischemic tissue (penumbra) by showing decreased cerebral blood flow (CBF),

increased mean transit time, and normal or increased cerebral blood volume (CBV)
- Infarcted tissue manifests with markedly decreased CBF and decreased CBV.
- Useful in acute management of patients who awaken with stroke symptoms.
- Requires use of contrast material

- **Magnetic resonance imaging (MRI)**
  - First done in 1977; uses intense magnetic images rather than radiation-like traditional radiographic studies.
  - **Diffusion-weighted imaging (DWI)**
    - Measures changes in diffusion properties of water in brain tissue
    - Restricted diffusion generally indicates unsalvageable brain tissue that is destined for infarction.
    - Accurate for detecting ischemia within minutes of occurrence
    - Differentiates acute infarcts from older infarcts
    - Does not require contrast material
  - **Magnetic resonance angiography (MRA)**
    - Similar to CTA; both the blood flow and the condition of the blood vessel walls can be seen.
    - Useful in detecting carotid artery dissection, intracranial aneurysms, and ateriovenous malformations (AVMs).
    - Does not require contrast material
  - **Magnetic resonance perfusion (MRP)**
    - Similar to CTP, it demonstrates CBF, mean transit time, and CBV.
    - Requires use of contrast material
  - **Magnetic resonance venography (MRV)**
    - Similar to MRA, but the technology is used only to visualize veins.
    - Requires use of contrast material

Perfusion–diffusion mismatch is utilized in acute stroke imaging to select patients for treatment beyond a strict 3-hour IV (intravenous) tissue plasminogen activator (tPA) time window. The difference between the diffusion (water content) of the tissue and perfusion (blood supply) abnormalities provides a measure of the ischemic penumbra. If the perfusion abnormality is larger than the area of restricted diffusion, the difference identifies the region of reversible ischemia that can be saved if blood flow is reestablished promptly.

POSITRON EMISSION TOMOGRAPHY (PET) SCAN

- Nuclear medicine-based technique that requires radioactive contrast, which raises the cost
  - For these two reasons it is not routinely used
- Most accurate method for measurement of regional cerebral perfusion and metabolism of glucose and oxygen

SINGLE PROTON EMISSION COMPUTED TOMOGRAPHY (SPECT) SCAN

- Useful in assessment of cerebral blood flow, vasoreactivity, and hemodynamic reserve
- Utilizes inhalation of carbon dioxide, or injection of acetazolamide, to induce vasodilatation of cerebral arterioles to stratify patients with carotid artery disease who may benefit from intervention.

CEREBRAL ANGIOGRAPHY—ALSO KNOWN AS DIGITAL SUBTRACTION ANGIOGRAPHY

- Visualization of blood vessels using fluoroscopy and contrast material
- Requires access through a large artery—usually the femoral artery; a catheter is threaded up past the heart to the cerebral vasculature.
- Standard against which all noninvasive assessments are compared

CAROTID DUPLEX

- Noninvasive ultrasound technology for assessment of carotid artery
- No contrast material used
- Lower sensitivity for detection of abnormality than CTA, MRA, or digital subtraction angiography (DSA)

TRANSCRANIAL DOPPLER (TCD)

- Noninvasive ultrasound technology for assessment of most large cerebral arteries (middle cerebral artery [MCA], anterior cerebral artery [ACA], carotid siphon, vertebral artery, basilar artery, ophthalmic artery)
- Approach is mainly via the temporal bone acoustic window (the area of thin bone above the zygomatic arch)
- Used to detect and quantify intracranial stenosis, occlusion, collateral flow, embolic events, and cerebral vasospasm (particularly after subarachnoid hemorrhage [SAH])
- Used to monitor the response to thrombolytic therapy

During clinical trials of TCD during thrombolytic therapy, it was noted that clot lysis was enhanced. This is apparently due to the effect of the ultrasonic energy agitating the clot, thus facilitating lysis. Numerous studies have been done but there has been no consensus. Many organizations continue to utilize TCD not just for monitoring, but also for augmentation of thrombolytic therapy.

LUMBAR PUNCTURE

- Used in cases of suspected SAH in which imaging does not show blood
- Cerebral spinal fluid (CSF) is analyzed for the presence of blood products; usually four tubes are extracted, as the presence of blood in the first or second tube may be due to the trauma of the procedure.
- Headache experienced by 10% to 30% of patients due to leakage of CSF from the dura.
  - Recent literature indicates that short duration (1 hour) of supine recumbence may be as efficient as long duration (4 hours) of supine recumbence to prevent headache.

ECHOCARDIOGRAPHY

- Cardioembolic sources are responsible for up to 30% of all strokes
- **Transthoracic (TTE)**
  - Done on all stroke patients
  - Excellent for identifying ventricular abnormalities such as dyskinetic wall segment
- **Transesophageal (TEE)**
  - Done on those patients in whom a cardiac source is strongly suspected

- Superior at identifying atrial and aortic abnormalities, such as patent foramen ovale or aortic arch atherosclerosis
- Requires passage of transducer catheter down the esophagus
- Visualization of the heart is superior because there is no impedance from chest muscles or the rib cage

ELECTROCARDIOGRAPHY

- Done on all stroke patients as part of the initial workup
- Used to identify atrial fibrillation, coexisting acute myocardial infarction (MI), cardiac arrhythmias, or chronic cardiac disease that may predispose to embolic sources

CHEST RADIOGRAPHY (CXR)

- May be done during the initial workup, but should not impede rapid evaluation and treatment decisions
- Valuable due to the high prevalence of cardiac disease in stroke patients

ELECTROENCEPHALOGRAM (EEG)

- Measures brain waves through several electrical leads attached to the scalp
- Not routinely used for stroke diagnosis, but may be done to rule out, or monitor, seizure activity

LABORATORY TESTS

- The only lab result that must precede the initiation of intravenous tPA is blood glucose and INR (international normalized ratio) for those patients on anticoagulation (Jauch et al., 2013).

- Blood glucose is often obtained through point-of-care finger stick, either by prehospital personnel or by emergency department personnel.
- Point-of-care INR can be done in many emergency departments.
  - Technology designed to check patients on anticoagulants, not as screening tool
  - Many hospital laboratories do not allow its use as overall INR screening tool
- All acute stroke patients should have:
  - Blood glucose, electrolytes, blood urea nitrogen (BUN), creatinine, complete blood count (CBC) with platelets, troponin, INR, partial thromboplastin time (PTT)
- Select patients may also have:
  - Liver function panel, toxicology screen, blood alcohol level, pregnancy test, HIV test, and arterial blood gas

7

Neurologic Assessment

In addition to understanding the anatomy and physiology of the brain, the ability to do a thorough neurologic assessment is another key skill of a neuroscience nurse. The combination of these abilities enables the neuroscience nurse to (a) correlate the findings on the assessment with the areas of the brain affected; (b) anticipate what changes to be vigilant for in the assessment over the next 24 to 48 hours.

The neurologic status of a patient with a new stroke can be expected to change frequently. Close monitoring is essential, but inconsistencies in terminology and assessment technique can make it difficult to track patient status. The use of standardized neurologic examination and documentation tools ensures that major components of the neurologic examination are accomplished efficiently and consistently. This consistency is critical not only in establishing a trend over time for each patient, but also in establishing population indicators for performance improvement efforts and for benchmarking.

In this chapter, you will learn:

1. The components of a neurologic assessment
2. A simple way to remember, and assess, the cranial nerves

STROKE-RELEVANT NEUROLOGIC ASSESSMENT

FAST FACTS in a NUTSHELL

It is important to differentiate a complete stroke-relevant neurologic assessment from a comprehensive neurologic examination in that the stroke-relevant assessment is focused on the brain and will be performed frequently during the hospital stay. Therefore, it is more abbreviated than the comprehensive examination, which includes all the cranial nerves (CN), reflexes, and spinal and peripheral nerve assessments.

- Starts at the head and progresses down to the feet
  - Level of consciousness and cognition—Includes the appropriateness of patient's responses, as well as orientation to person, place, and time
  - Pupils—Size, symmetry, reactivity to light, and whether consistent with prior exam; abnormality indicates CN II involvement
  - Extraocular movements—Range of motion of the eyes; gaze palsy; abnormality indicates CN III, IV, or VI involvement
  - Fields of vision—Checking for field cuts or loss of vision in a portion of the visual field; abnormality indicates CN III, IV, or VI involvement, or visual extinction (parietal lobe involvement)
  - Facial symmetry—Checking for facial droop; loss of nasolabial fold is subtle indication of droop; abnormality is due to motor fiber involvement or CN V involvement

- Speech—Checking for clarity (abnormality is dysarthria) and for ability to use language to communicate, either in expression or in understanding; also referred to as reception (abnormality is aphasia). Abnormalities are due to speech area involvement.
- Swallow ability—Abnormality is due to motor fiber involvement.
- Arm and leg strength—Abnormalities are due to motor fiber involvement, either cortical (motor strip) or subcortical (basal ganglia).
- Coordination and balance—Ataxia is utilized in most assessments; abnormalities are due to cerebellar involvement.
- Sensation—Testing ability to feel a stimulation (pin prick, firm touch, noxious stimuli for minimally conscious, or unconscious patient) as well as comparing right to left side (patient's eyes are closed); abnormality is due to sensory fiber involvement, either cortical (sensory strip) or subcortical (basal ganglia).
- Extinction—Can be tactile, visual, auditory, or spatial; characterized by an inability to be aware of a stimulation when presented simultaneously on right and left sides; abnormality is due to right parietal lobe involvement.
  - Tactile: Assessment is accomplished during the sensation assessment by applying stimulation simultaneously to both sides (patient's eyes are closed). If the patient had reported normal sensation when each side had been individually stimulated, but then only reports feeling one side when simultaneously stimulated, the patient has tactile extinction.
  - Visual: Assessment is accomplished during visual field assessment by presenting visual stimulation simultaneously to both sides.
  - Auditory: Assessment is accomplished by providing simultaneous sound stimulation to both ears.
  - Spatial: Assessment is accomplished by (a) asking the patient to describe what he or she sees in his or

her surroundings; (b) observing the patient's eating pattern (does he or she only eat the right side of the plate of food?); (c) having the patient read (does he or she only read the right half of the page?) or (d) having the patient draw a clock (does he or she only draw the right side of the clock face?).

- Proprioception—Checking the ability to be aware of one's body position within the environment; tested by having patient close the eyes, then moving his or her finger or toe, and asking the patient what position that digit is now in; abnormality is due to parietal lobe involvement.
- The National Institutes of Health Stroke Scale (NIHSS) is discussed in Chapter 8 (see Figure 8.1).

FAST FACTS in a NUTSHELL

A simple way to remember where each speech area is located and its specific function is by looking at the first vowels in the words: Broca's area is in the frontal lobe and controls motor speech; Wernicke's area is in the temporal lobe and controls receptive speech.

- The assessment schedule varies by organization but it is generally accepted to be according to care level:
  - ICU (intensive care unit)—hourly
  - Transitional or intermediate care unit—every 2 hours
  - General neuroscience unit—every 4 hours
  - There are specific requirements for IV tPA and acute intervention patients.
- With a paper system, flowsheets and tables are utilized that facilitate easy visualization of trends, but necessitate a manual process for utilization of data for population analysis.

- With electronic medical records (EMR), assessment is documented into individual fields that can be exported into tables and graphs for analysis, but makes visualization of trends quite challenging.

======================*FAST FACTS in a NUTSHELL*

There are many mnemonics to help us remember the names of the 12 cranial nerves: olfactory, optic, oculomotor, trochlear, trigeminal, abducens, facial, acoustic, glossopharyngeal, vagus, accessory, hypoglossal. One of the most common—and socially acceptable—is *On Old Olympus Towering Top a Finn and German Viewed a Hops*. But how do we remember what each of them does? The answer is the Cranial Nerve Face (Figure 7.1; Bolek, 2006).

- Cranial nerve assessment can seem daunting, and has been identified as a barrier to nurses working in neuroscience roles. Below are some practical tips to allow assessment of the cranial nerves in a few minutes.

Cranial Nerve	Testing Technique
1 Olfactory	Can you smell this? Use coffee or mint
2 Optic	Can you see this? Snellen chart or visual confrontation
3 Oculomotor	Follow my finger, testing extraocular movement (EOM)
4 Trochlear	Look down
5 Trigeminal	Facial sensation, clench the teeth, corneal reflex
6 Abducens	Look out to the side

(continued)

(*continued*)

Cranial Nerve	Testing Technique
7 Facial	Smile, raise your eyebrows
8 Acoustic	Can you hear this? Crinkle paper at the ear
9 Glossopharyngeal	Intact gag and swallow reflex
10 Vagus	Hoarse? Open up and say "ahh"
11 Spinal accessory	Shrug the shoulders
12 Hypoglossal	Stick out the tongue, look for deviation

Cranial nerves by the numbers

The next time you're trying to remember the locations and functions of the cranial nerves, picture this drawing. All 12 cranial nerves are represented, though some may be a little harder to spot than others. For example, the shoulders are formed by the number "11" because cranial nerve XI controls neck and shoulder movement. If you immediately recognize that the sides of the face and the top of the head are formed by the number "7," you're well on your way to using this memory device.

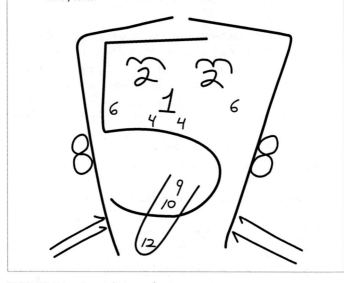

FIGURE 7.1 Cranial nerve face.
Source: Copyright © 2013, HealthCom Media. All rights reserved. *American Nurse Today*, November 2006, www.AmericanNurseToday.com

8

Stroke Severity Scores

Quality indicators such as mortality rate, complication rate, and length of stay have been difficult to compare among comprehensive stroke centers, primary stroke centers, and all other hospitals without essential details about the severity of the stroke. Comprehensive stroke centers, by design, will care for the most complex stroke patients who may not meet the criteria for higher "severity of illness" under the current system. Therefore, when unadjusted outcomes are compared, comprehensive centers may appear to provide inferior care due to higher complication and mortality rates in the more complex patients.

Clinically, the use of standardized severity scores provides an efficient, consistent assessment method that produces a score that can be utilized in hand-off reports and in daily progress monitoring.

In this chapter, you will learn:

1. The various severity scores utilized for different types of stroke

NIH STROKE SCALE	Neuro A&P Correlation
Level of Consciousness (LOC): 0 = Alert 1 = Drowsy 2 = Obtunded 3 = Unresponsive	LOC
LOC to Questions: *Ask patient month and age* 0 = Both correct 1 = One correct 2 = Neither correct	LOC
LOC to Commands: *Open, close eyes; make fist, let go; substitute other one step command if needed* 0 = Obeys both correctly 1 = Obeys one correctly 2 = Neither correct	LOC
Best Gaze: *Eyes open, patient follows examiner's fingers or face horizontally. Only test horizontal gaze.* 0 = Normal 1 = Partial gaze palsy 2 = Forced deviation	CN III, VI
Visual: *Face patient, hold hand out at edge of visual field, display 1, 2, or 5 fingers. Have patient report how many fingers he or she sees. Do this in all 4 visual-field quadrants. Use your visual field as baseline for normal. Alternative: wiggle finger at edge of visual field and bring in until patient sees it.* 0 = No visual loss 1 = Partial hemianopsia 3 = Bilateral hemianopsia	CN II
Facial Palsy: *Show teeth, raise eyebrows, and squeeze eyes shut* 0 = Normal 1 = Minor asymmetry 2 = Partial (lower face paralysis) 3 = Complete unilateral paralysis	CN VII/ Motor
Motor Arm—Left: *Elevate extremity 45 degrees for 10 seconds and score drift movement.* 0 = No drift 1 = Drift before 10 seconds 2 = Falls before 10 seconds 3 = No effort against gravity (falls immediately) 4 = No movement	Motor

FIGURE 8.1 NIHSS score sheet.
Adapted from NINDS NIHSS: http://www.ninds nih.gov/doctors/NIH_stroke_scale.pdf

NIH STROKE SCALE	Neuro A&P Correlation
Motor Arm—Right: *Elevate extremity 45 degrees for 10 seconds and score drift / movement.* 0 = No drift 1 = Drift before 10 seconds 2 = Falls before 10 seconds 3 = No effort against gravity (falls immediately) 4 = No movement	Motor
Motor Leg—Left: *Elevate extremity 30 degrees for 5 seconds and score drift / movement.* 0 = No drift 1 = Drift before 5 seconds 2 = Falls before 5 seconds 3 = No effort against gravity (falls immediately) 4 = No movement	Motor
Motor Leg—Right: *Elevate extremity 30 degrees for 5 seconds and score drift / movement.* 0 = No drift 1 = Drift before 5 seconds 2 = Falls before 5 seconds 3 = No effort against gravity (falls immediately) 4 = No movement	Motor
Limb Ataxia: *Finger to nose: Hold your finger up for patient to see, have patient take his or her finger and touch his or her nose, then touch your finger, and repeat a few times. Heel down shin: Help patient place heel of unaffected side on upper shin of affected side and slide heel down shin. Do same on both sides. Score only if inability to perform task is out of proportion to patient's weakness. If score > 1 on motor, do not score ataxia for that limb.* 0 = Absent 1 = Present in upper **or** lower 2 = Present in both upper and lower	Cerebellar
Sensory: *Sensation or grimace to pinprick to face, arm, trunk, and leg compared side to side. Use proximal portion of limbs. Score only sensory loss attributable to stroke, not pre-existing loss (diabetic neuropathy, etc.) Alternative method: use cold sensation like metal of stethoscope, pen, penlight, etc.* 0 = Normal 1 = Mild—Pt feels pinprick/coldness but it is dull compared to other side 2 = Patient not aware of being touched	Sensory

FIGURE 8.1 NIHSS score sheet (*continued*).
Adapted from NINDS NIHSS: http://www.ninds.nih.gov/doctors/NIH_stroke_scale.pdf

NIH STROKE SCALE	Neuro A&P Correlation
Best Language: *Name items, describe a picture or read sentences. Can have patient name simple items like pen, neck tie, glasses, TV, etc.; looking for inability to name objects or inability to comprehend.* 0 = No aphasia 1 = Mild to moderate aphasia 2 = Severe aphasia 3 = Mute	Speech/language
Dysarthria: *Evaluate speech clarity by patient repeating words; ask intubated patients to write words.* *Suggested words: Mama Tip-top Fifty-fifty* *Thanks Huckleberry Baseball player* *Sentences: You know how. Down to earth. I got home from work. Near the table in the dining room.* 0 = Normal articulation 1 = Mild to moderate slurring—can be understood with some difficulty 2 = Severe—near unintelligible or mute	Cerebellar
Extinction and Inattention (Neglect): *Have patient close eyes. Touch one side at a time, have patient indicate which side is being touched. Touch both sides simultaneously and assess patient's response. Next, hold hands out at edge of visual fields, wiggle fingers, have patient say when he or she sees fingers wiggle.* 0 = Normal, no neglect 1 = Partial neglect (mild hemi-attention) 2 = Profound neglect (does not recognize stimulation, or orients to only one side)	Sensory

Key: Score 1-5: anticipate discharge to home—patient may require outpatient services
        6–13: anticipate discharge to acute rehab
      > 13: anticipate discharge to extended care facility
<div align="right">**TOTAL SCORE:**</div>	

FIGURE 8.1   NIHSS score sheet (*continued*).
Adapted from NINDS NIHSS: http://www.ninds nih.gov/doctors/NIH_stroke_scale.pdf

NATIONAL INSTITUTES OF HEALTH STROKE SCALE (NIHSS)

- Created in 1983 by the National Institute for Neurological Diseases and Stroke (NINDS; Figure 8.1)
  - Initially utilized to determine candidacy for inclusion in stroke research trials
  - Range of score is 0 to 42; points are earned for deficit: the higher the score, the greater the deficits
- Standardized language for describing stroke deficit
- Utilized for both ischemic and hemorrhagic stroke patients
- Predicts severity of injury and correlates with patient outcome
  - 80% of patients with an NIHSS less than 12 to 14 have good or excellent outcome; 20% of patients with an NIHSS greater than 20 to 26 have good or excellent outcome
  - NIHSS score greater than 22 on admission has 17% higher risk of hemorrhagic conversion after administration of intravenous tissue plasminogen activator
- Predicts discharge disposition
  - NIHSS less than 5 indicates likely discharge to home
  - NIHSS of 6 to 13 indicates likely discharge to acute rehabilitation facility
  - NIHSS greater than 13 indicates likely discharge to nursing home or heaven
- Utility of admission and discharge scores
  - Calculation of change reflects effect of stroke and progress/deterioration in individual patients
  - Population scores—mean, median, range—are representative of each stroke type outcome
- Modified NIHSS (mNIHSS)
  - Derived from the original NIHSS
  - Eliminated redundancy and poorly reliable items:
    - Level of consciousness (felt to be redundant), facial palsy, ataxia, dysarthria
  - Score range 0 to 31
  - Reliability tested to be superior to the NIHSS, but NIHSS continues to be used more often

FAST FACTS in a NUTSHELL

Although studies have shown that an increase or decrease of 4 points in the stroke score indicates important changes in the patient's neurological status, it is the content of the neurological exam changes that determines the necessity for notification of the provider. Therefore, nursing care protocols should not base notification of the provider on the 4-point-change alone. A patient with loss of arm strength, with no other changes, will only have an increase of 3 points, but warrants action by the health care team.

INTRACEREBRAL HEMORRHAGE SCORES

Original ICH (intracerebral hemorrhage) score (ICH) and modified ICH score (mICH) (Table 8.1)

- Utilized for ICH patients (Cheung & Liang-Yu, 2013)
- Research has found the ICH and mICH are equivalent in predicting outcomes
- Recent research suggests that a score at 24-hours post-hemorrhage is more accurate than admission score

TABLE 8.1 ICH Score Components

ICH	mICH

Glascow Coma Scale
  3–4 = 2 points
  5–12 = 1 point
  13–15 = 0 points
	NIHSS

Age > 80 = 1 point	Admission temperature
ICH volume ≥ 30 = 1 point	Pulse pressure
IVH = 1 point	IVH
Infratentorial origin of hemorrhage = 1 point	Subarachnoid extension of hemorrhage

IVH, intraventricular hemorrhage.

- **Hunt and Hess Score (Table 8.2)**
  - Most commonly used severity scale for the subarachnoid hemorrhage (SAH) population (Rosen & MacDonald, 2005)
  - Based on patient's level of consciousness and accompanying symptoms
  - Initially established for surgical risk prediction
  - 80% correlation with outcomes at 6 months poststroke

TABLE 8.2 Hunt and Hess Score Components

1. Asymptomatic, mild headache, slight nuchal rigidity
2. Moderate to severe headache, nuchal rigidity, no neurologic deficit other than cranial nerve palsy
3. Drowsiness/confusion, mild focal neurologic deficit
4. Stupor, moderate to severe hemiparesis
5. Coma, decerebrate posturing

- **Fisher Scale Score (Table 8.3)**
  - Established in 1980 to predict cerebral vasospasm after SAH (Rosen & MacDonald, 2005)
  - Based on amount/location of blood present on initial CT scan
  - Correlation to outcomes has been demonstrated

TABLE 8.3 Fisher Scale Score Components

1. No hemorrhage evident
2. SAH less than 1-mm thick
3. SAH more than 1-mm thick
4. SAH of any thickness with intraventricular hemorrhage or parenchymal extension

- **World Federation of Neurological Surgeons (WFNS) Score (Table 8.4)**
  - Established in 1988 as a clinical severity grading tool (Rosen & MacDonald, 2005)

TABLE 8.4 WFNS Score Components

Grade	GCS	Motor deficit
I	15	–
II	14–13	–
III	14–13	+
IV	12–7	+/–
V	6–3	+/–

- Based on Glasgow Coma Scale score and presence/absence of motor deficit
- Correlation to outcomes is less well demonstrated than Hunt and Hess

- **Glasgow Coma Scale**
  - Established in 1974 to evaluate depth of decreased consciousness and coma in head-injury population
  - Range of score is 0 to 15, with points deducted for deficit; the higher the score, the better the patient status.

FAST FACTS in a NUTSHELL

The GCS has become a common method for measuring the level of consciousness in the neuroscience population. It is quick and simple to score; however, its application in the stroke population is limited. The rules for scoring the motor response are to score the "best response," so a patient with a hemiplegia who is awake could earn a "perfect" 15, while unable to move half the body.

ABCD2 SCORE

- Acronym stands for Age, Blood pressure, Clinical features, Duration of symptoms, and Diabetes.

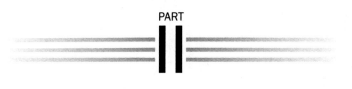

PART

II

Saving the Penumbra

9

Acute Ischemic Stroke Interventions

Considering how long the medical community has known what a stroke is, acute interventions are still in their infancy. Tissue plasminogen activator (tPA) was approved by the Food and Drug Administration (FDA) in 1996, and the first endovascular intervention, the MERCI Retrieval Device, was approved by the FDA in 2004. Other endovascular devices that are described in this chapter have been approved in the years since 2004, but tPA remains the only drug approved by the FDA for acute stroke intervention. It is not without controversy, even 17 years later, but numerous studies have demonstrated its safety when guidelines are followed, even in the cases of stroke mimics or mild/improving strokes.

The endovascular mechanical interventions were approved by the FDA on the basis of their ability to remove clots, not necessarily because of improved outcomes of patients—a decision that has also been considered controversial by some experts. The effectiveness of the endovascular devices has improved with each new product, and when guidelines are followed—and with careful patient selection—these devices provide a valuable option for treatment of large vessel occlusions.

In this chapter, you will learn:

1. The basis of, and controversy around, the FDA approval of intravenous (IV) tPA
2. The endovascular interventions—their differences and similarities

tPA: GIVEN INTRAVENOUSLY

- Initially approved for use in myocardial infarction (MI) and massive pulmonary embolus
- Studies that contributed to FDA approval:
  - Protocol for the Evaluation of Tissue Plasminogen Activator Early in the Course of Acute Stroke
    - Small pilot study done to evaluate safety
    - Used in design of National Institute of Neurological Diseases and Stroke (NINDS) study
- NINDS tPA Stroke Trial
  - Two-part study: Part I, 291 patients; part II, 333 patients
  - Demonstrated 30% better functional outcomes at 3 months posttreatment compared to similar populations not treated, as well as a higher intracerebral hemorrhage (ICH) rate
  - Analysis results were that benefits outweighed incidence of ICH
  - European Cooperative Acute Stroke Study (ECASS), 620 patients
  - Dose was 22% higher than NINDS study dose
  - Demonstrated higher ICH and mortality rate than those not treated
  - Provided evidence of need for maximum dose of 90 mg regardless of patient weight
  - Thrombolytic Therapy of Acute Thrombotic/Thrombolytic Stroke Study (TTATTS), 24 patients
  - Demonstrated higher ICH rates with treatment window of 6 hours from stroke onset
  - Provided evidence of need for time limitations for administration

As a result of the numerous studies done, IV tPA was approved with a dose restriction of 90 mg, time restriction of 3 hours from symptom onset, and an extensive list of exclusion criteria. Since 1996, some of the exclusion criteria have come to be considered as relative criteria, meaning that the provider decides on a case-specific basis.

- Professional organizations of emergency department physicians initially took a stand against tPA
- The American Academy of Emergency Medicine (AAEM)
  - 2002 Position Statement: The evidence used as the basis for FDA approval was insufficient to warrant it being considered a "standard of care"; the results of the research could not be duplicated in the average hospital, so they would not support its use
  - 2012 Position Statement: Sixteen years after the FDA decision, an independent, structured review was conducted by two emergency medicine physicians. They found that:
    1. tPA is safe and effective for acute ischemic stroke
    2. Early thrombolytic treatment of stroke improves outcomes in acute ischemic stroke
    3. tPA administered 3 to 4.5 hours after acute ischemic stroke improves outcomes without increasing mortality (DeMers et al., 2012)
- The American College of Emergency Physicians (ACEP)
  - 2002 Position Statement: "IV tPA may be an efficacious therapy but there is insufficient evidence to endorse the use of tPA when systems are not in place to insure that NINDS guidelines are followed" (Donnell, 2009, p. 296).
  - 2012 Policy Statement in collaboration with the American Academy of Neurology (AAN): IV tPA is safe and effective for acute ischemic stroke within 3 hours and within 3 to 4.5 hours for select patients (Edlow et al., 2013)

Tissue plasminogen activator does not work for all stroke patients; in fact, rarely are there dramatic improvements witnessed after administering the medication. The results are more subtle, only evident after discharge, adding to the challenge for acute care nurses to appreciate its impact.

- Administration Guide
  - Dosage calculation: 0.9 mg/kg infused over 1 hour; 10% of dose to be administered as initial bolus over 1 minute
  - Total dose must never exceed 90 mg regardless of patient weight
  - Complications to monitor for: angioedema, systemic bleeding, anaphylaxis
  - Vital sign and neurologic checks documentation schedule:
    - Every 15 min × 2 hours (starting at infusion), then
    - Every 30 min × 6 hours, then
    - Every hour × 16 hours, then according to level of care

Endovascular Interventions

Approach is via femoral artery with the device threaded up past the heart, into the major cerebral arteries

- Vital sign and neurologic checks documentation schedule is same as above, starting at the end of the procedure.

Intra-arterial (IA) tPA

- Time frame of tPA administration is 6 hours from symptom onset.
- Not approved by the FDA; IMS III (Interventional Management of Stroke) trial did not show superiority over IV tPA alone, which is much less invasive; but is used widely as "offlabel," with written consent.

SUBARACHNOID HEMORRHAGE SCORES

- **Hunt and Hess Score (Table 8.2)**
  - Most commonly used severity scale for the sub-arachnoid hemorrhage (SAH) population (Rosen & MacDonald, 2005)
  - Based on patient's level of consciousness and accompanying symptoms
  - Initially established for surgical risk prediction
  - 80% correlation with outcomes at 6 months poststroke

TABLE 8.2 Hunt and Hess Score Components

1. Asymptomatic, mild headache, slight nuchal rigidity
2. Moderate to severe headache, nuchal rigidity, no neurologic deficit other than cranial nerve palsy
3. Drowsiness/confusion, mild focal neurologic deficit
4. Stupor, moderate to severe hemiparesis
5. Coma, decerebrate posturing

- **Fisher Scale Score (Table 8.3)**
  - Established in 1980 to predict cerebral vasospasm after SAH (Rosen & MacDonald, 2005)
  - Based on amount/location of blood present on initial CT scan
  - Correlation to outcomes has been demonstrated

TABLE 8.3 Fisher Scale Score Components

1. No hemorrhage evident
2. SAH less than 1-mm thick
3. SAH more than 1-mm thick
4. SAH of any thickness with intraventricular hemorrhage or parenchymal extension

- **World Federation of Neurological Surgeons (WFNS) Score (Table 8.4)**
  - Established in 1988 as a clinical severity grading tool (Rosen & MacDonald, 2005)

TABLE 8.4 WFNS Score Components

Grade	GCS	Motor deficit
I	15	−
II	14–13	−
III	14–13	+
IV	12–7	+/−
V	6–3	+/−

- Based on Glasgow Coma Scale score and presence/absence of motor deficit
- Correlation to outcomes is less well demonstrated than Hunt and Hess

- **Glasgow Coma Scale**
  - Established in 1974 to evaluate depth of decreased consciousness and coma in head-injury population
  - Range of score is 0 to 15, with points deducted for deficit; the higher the score, the better the patient status.

FAST FACTS in a NUTSHELL

The GCS has become a common method for measuring the level of consciousness in the neuroscience population. It is quick and simple to score; however, its application in the stroke population is limited. The rules for scoring the motor response are to score the "best response," so a patient with a hemiplegia who is awake could earn a "perfect" 15, while unable to move half the body.

ABCD2 SCORE

- Acronym stands for <u>A</u>ge, <u>B</u>lood pressure, <u>C</u>linical features, <u>D</u>uration of symptoms, and <u>D</u>iabetes.

- Established for predicting short-term risk of stroke in patients with transient ischemic attack (TIA; 7 days post TIA; Johnston et al., 2007)
- Effective in distinguishing true TIAs from mimics such as dizziness and altered level of consciousness
- Utilized in the emergency department to determine whether admission is advised (score 4 or above), or discharge with outpatient workup (score less than 4)
- Range of score is 0 to 7 (Table 8.5)
  - 1 to 3 = low risk
  - 4 to 5 = moderate risk
  - 6 to 7 = high risk

TABLE 8.5 ABCD2 Score Components

Age > 60 years	1
Elevated blood pressure (BP) systolic ≥ 140; diastolic ≥ 90	1
Diabetes	1
Unilateral weakness	2
Speech impairment	1
Symptom duration	
> 60 min	2
10–59 min	1
< 10 min	0
Total possible score	7

- Success of newer mechanical retrieval devices has diminished the efficacy of IA administration alone.
- Mainly utilized as adjunct to mechanical retrieval; infused after clot removal to "clean up," or dissolve, any residual clots.

Mechanical Retrieval Devices

- Time frame of procedure is 8 hours from symptom onset.
- MERCI Retrieval Device—Mechanical Embolus Removal in Cerebral Ischemia
  - Corkscrew device that is advanced past the clot and, when withdrawn, engages with the clot and pulls it out.
  - Recanalization (vessel reopening) success reported as 48% to 59%
    - Success dependent on ability to pass the device beyond the clot
    - Not uncommon for clot to be disrupted, with partial success in removal; IA tPA then infused
  - FDA approval in 2004
  - Seldom utilized anymore, having been replaced by the Penumbra System and the newer stent retrieval systems
- Penumbra System
  - Clot disruption and suction device in which a "separator" is threaded through the suction device and used to disrupt the clot. As pieces are broken loose, they are pulled back into the suction catheter. This process is repeated until the clot is removed.
  - Recanalization success rate reported as 52% to 86%
  - FDA approval in 2008
- Stent Retrievers: Solitaire and Trevo Devices
  - Mechanism is a self-expanding, stent-like device inserted into the blockage through a sheath. Once the sheath is through the clot, it is withdrawn, releasing the stent, which expands, compressing the clot against the arterial wall. After several minutes (time allowed for the clot to become more engaged

with the stent filaments), the device is collapsed and withdrawn, pulling the clot with it
- Recanalization success rates reported as 70% to 92%
- Solitaire Flow Restoration (FR) approved by the FDA in 2012
- Trevo Pro Retriever approved by the FDA in 2012, a few months after Solitaire was approved
- Acute Angioplasty and Stenting
  - Increasingly being done for intracranial and extra-cranial carotid or vertebral arteries in two specific situations:
    - When the primary cause of the stroke is attenuation or cessation of flow, as with severe atherosclerosis or dissection
    - When catheter access to an intracranial thrombus is impeded by severe stenosis of the extracranial carotid
  - There are no completed prospective, randomized controlled trials as yet, but small retrospective case series have reported promising results.

FAST FACTS in a NUTSHELL

Numerous clinical trials have been conducted, and many are currently in progress, seeking more options for acute ischemic stroke intervention. The challenge going forward will be to enroll patients—in the midst of their acute stroke emergency—into a clinical trial when there are proven therapies available. By agreeing to the clinical trial, the patient is accepting the possibility of being assigned to the "control group," meaning no acute intervention is done; even if they get assigned to the "intervention group," it is only an investigational treatment, not a proven one.

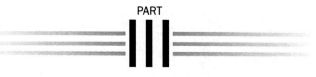

PART

III

Mechanical Interventions
for Secondary Prevention

10

Ischemic Stroke

Key components of acute ischemic stroke care are geared toward recanalization, stabilization, and saving the penumbra. Less obvious, but equally important, components of acute ischemic stroke care focus on secondary stroke prevention. Valiant efforts by the health care team can be rendered useless if the patient suffers another stroke as a result of risk factors that were not addressed with acute interventions. Most of the diagnostic tests that are performed during the initial hospital stay are done to determine the etiology, or cause, of the stroke. Why do we want to know the cause? So that we can customize the care plan to prevent a second stroke . . . secondary prevention. Many of the risk factors cannot be fixed quickly, but those that can, should be. The medical management of risk factors for secondary prevention will be discussed in Chapter 17.

In this chapter, you will learn:

1. Clinical trial phases (Table 10.1)—what do they represent?
2. The background and clinical application of the TOAST (Trial of ORG 10172 in Acute Stroke Treatment) criteria

3. The pros and cons of carotid endarterectomy and carotid stenting
4. Patent foramen ovale (PFO) management
5. Hemicraniectomy—What does this do for secondary prevention?

TABLE 10.1 Clinical Trial Phases

Phase I	• Assesses the safety of a drug/device • Can take several months • Usually involves a small number of healthy volunteers (20 to 100), who are paid • Determines the effects of the drug/device on humans • Also investigates side effects that occur as dosage levels are increased • 70% of experimental drugs pass this phase of testing
Phase II	• Assesses the efficacy of a drug/device • Can last from several months to 2 years • Involves up to several hundred patients • Most are randomized trials—one group of patients receives the experimental drug, while a second "control" group receives a standard treatment or placebo • Often "blinded," which means that neither the patients nor the researchers know who has received the experimental drug • One third of experimental drugs successfully complete this phase
Phase III	• Involves randomized and blind testing in several hundred to several thousand patients • Can last several years • Thorough evaluation of the effectiveness of the drug or device, the benefits and the range of possible adverse reactions • 70% to 90% of drugs successfully complete this phase of testing • Pharmaceutical company can request Food and Drug Administration (FDA) approval for marketing the drug
Phase IV	• Often called postmarketing surveillance trials • Conducted after a drug or device has been approved for consumer sale

(continued)

TABLE 10.1 Clinical Trial Phases (continued)

- Pharmaceutical company's objectives: (1) Compare a drug with other drugs already in the market; (2) monitor a drug's long-term effectiveness and impact on a patient's quality of life; and (3) determine the cost-effectiveness of a drug therapy relative to other traditional and new therapies
- Can result in a drug or device being taken off the market or restrictions of use being placed on the product

FAST FACTS in a NUTSHELL

Stroke research lingo can be intimidating. Understanding some key terms can help us to understand what is being stated. For instance, what do they mean when they say that they are testing for efficacy versus safety? There is an important distinction; both are very important, but one without the other is useless.

Safety: Is the treatment/drug safe? = Does it cause harm?

Efficacy: Does the treatment/drug work? = Does the drug/device do what you want it to do?

TOAST CRITERIA (TRIAL OF ORG 10172 IN ACUTE STROKE TREATMENT)

- Classification system developed for a research study, published in 1993
- Five categories of subtypes based on the etiology of strokes (Adams et al., 1993)
  - Large-artery atherosclerosis (embolus/thrombosis)
  - Cardioembolism (high risk/medium risk)
  - Small-vessel occlusion (lacune)
  - Stroke of other determined etiology

- Stroke of undetermined etiology
  - Two or more causes identified
  - Negative evaluation
  - Incomplete evaluation
- Original intention of the TOAST criteria was for management of secondary prevention; by identifying the etiology, treatment and focused risk-factor reduction would facilitate prevention of subsequent strokes
- Recent research has demonstrated that the TOAST criteria continues to be relevant—not just in identification of etiology, but also in stratification of vascular risk
  - Large-artery atherosclerosis and cardioembolism have higher risk of secondary stroke than the other subtypes

LARGE-ARTERY ATHEROSCLEROSIS MANAGEMENT

- Emboli composed of cholesterol crystals dislodged from the atheromatous plaques situated on the aorta and the carotid and vertebral–basilar arteries are common.
- Aortic plaques increase the risk of stroke during cardiopulmonary bypass surgery and cardiac catheterization.

CAROTID ENDARTERECTOMY (CEA)

- First performed in 1953
- Indicated for symptomatic carotid stenosis with greater than 60% loss of lumen, or asymptomatic high-grade carotid stenosis with greater than 70% loss of lumen
- Three major trials have consistently demonstrated that patients with less than 50% stenosis did not benefit from intervention.
- Benefit is highest if done during the initial 2 weeks after the transient ischemic attack (TIA) or mild stroke for neurologically stable patients.

CAROTID ARTERY STENTING (CAS)

- Reported in 1980, approved by the Food and Drug Administration in 2004 amid great controversy
  - Indicated for symptomatic, high-risk patients with greater than 70% stenosis
  - Turf battle between experienced surgeons performing carotid endarterectomy (CEA), and less experienced nonsurgical specialists performing carotid artery stenting (CAS)
  - Improvements in technology as well as in training/ experience of providers have led to greater professional acceptance of this treatment option.
- Benefits are no need for anesthesia, no surgical incision, shorter hospital stay
  - Best option for patients with extensive comorbidities that make surgery unadvisable

CARDIOEMBOLISM MANAGEMENT

Atrial Fibrillation

- One of the most prevalent causes of stroke and TIA, particularly as people get older
- Left Atrial Appendage Occlusion Device
  - Endovascular placement
  - Research is ongoing; early results indicate efficacy similar to that of medical management with warfarin
  - Clinical utility likely will be in patients at high risk for stroke who are poor candidates for medical management with anticoagulants
- Cardioversion
  - Indicated for symptomatic atrial fibrillation (aFib or AF; acute dyspnea or heart failure symptoms)
  - Must be confident of new onset and that there is no clot present in heart—transesophageal echocardiography (TEE)
  - Not indicated in the acute phase of stroke management

FAST FACTS in a NUTSHELL

> Older people are more prone to atrial fibrillation since the myocardium tends to stretch with age and with long-standing hypertension. With stretching, the electrical conduction of the impulse between the sinoatrial (SA) node and the atrioventricular (AV) node is interrupted, and atrial fibrillation is triggered.

Patent Foramen Ovale

- Present in up to 25% of the adult population
- Patent foramen ovale (PFO) was detected in cryptogenic stroke more often in younger patients: 43.9% versus 28.3% in older patients
- The presence of PFO seen on echocardiogram should trigger two actions:
  - TEE to facilitate better visualization
  - Thorough assessment for possibility of deep vein thrombosis (DVT)
- Numerous research studies have been done with no clear recommendation for closure over medical management with antiplatelets or anticoagulants
  - Many insurance providers do not cover the cost of PFO closure
  - Size of the PFO, and the presence of atrial–septal aneurysm, are variables that have made clear recommendations elusive
  - Difficult for young patients as long-term anticoagulation creates limitations related to occupation and leisure activities
- PFO closure devices: surgical and endovascular
  - Majority of studies have demonstrated low complication rates and outcomes that are superior to medical management (low 3-year recurrent event rate).

Question: What physical condition must be present in order for a DVT to cause a stroke? *Answer:* PFO. A DVT that becomes mobile will normally travel through the vena cava into the right side of the heart and pass through the pulmonary veins to the lungs, causing pulmonary embolus (PE). If a PFO is present, it creates a "doorway" for a clot to cross from the right side of the heart to the left, enabling it to pass through the aorta and up to the brain, causing stroke (Figure 10.1).

Hemicraniectomy

- Involves excision of scalp and temporary removal of a piece of the cranium
  - Size is generally 12 cm (anterior–posterior) by 9 cm (superior–inferior)
  - Meninges are stretched back into place, and the scalp is sutured closed over the top

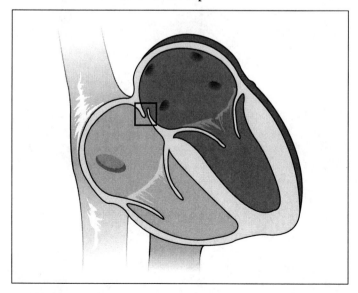

FIGURE 10.1 Patent foramen ovale.

- The "bone flap" is either stored in subcutaneous tissue of the abdomen, or stored in the freezer, or discarded and artificial material is used for replacement.
- Replacement is done at 6 to 8 weeks.
- Indicated for large-volume infarctions (hemispheric or cerebellar) in patients less than 60 years of age.
- Outcomes are reduced mortality and reduced incidence of secondary ischemic stroke.
  - Mortality rate is reduced from 78% to 29% in clinical trials.
  - High intracranial pressure produces brainstem compression, with secondary involvement of the frontal and occipital lobes. Compression of the anterior cerebral and posterior cerebral arteries against dural structures results in secondary ischemic stroke.

11

Hemorrhagic Stroke

Mechanical intervention for secondary prevention of hemorrhagic stroke looks very different from the clot retrieval systems used for ischemic stroke. But, similar to the ischemic interventions, there have been turf wars among neurosurgery, neurology, and neuro-endovascular interventional professionals as to what is the best treatment, who should perform the intervention, and when is the best time to intervene. Numerous studies have been conducted, along with one very large multicenter, randomized subarachnoid hemorrhage (SAH) trial designed to answer these questions. There was consensus that a team approach to selecting the best therapeutic option for each patient is necessary. Standards for Comprehensive Stroke Center certification echo this opinion, and require institutions to demonstrate that their practitioners consult professional colleagues for treatment decisions. In addition, the experience and expertise of the practitioners (measured by the number of cases per year) should be a minimum of 10 per year.

Some of the acute interventions for hemorrhagic stroke are focused on control of intracranial pressure

(continued)

> *(continued)*
>
> *and prevention of complications such as hydrocephalus—secondary prevention of ischemic stroke, not hemorrhagic stroke. Interventions such as intraventricular thrombolysis, external ventricular drain (EVD), and shunts are described in this chapter.*

In this chapter, you will learn:

1. Recommendations for selection of treatment options for aneurysmal subarachnoid hemorrhage (aSAH) and arteriovenous malformations (AVMs)
2. Indications for surgical evacuation of intracerebral hematoma (ICH)
3. Intraventricular thrombolysis: Do we really give clot buster to patients with brain bleeds?

ANEURYSM OBLITERATION

Aneurysm therapy is designed to isolate the aneurysm or reduce the arterial pressure within it, to strengthen the walls by encasing the material around it, or to promote thrombosis in it.

- Intervention should be done as early as feasible to reduce the risk of rebleeding, preferably within the first 72 hours (Connolly et al., 2012).
  - Risk of rebleed is highest within first 24 hours.
- Ruptured aneurysms, judged amenable to both surgical clipping and endovascular coiling, should be coiled.
- Patients with large (> 50 mL) ICH and middle cerebral artery (MCA) aneurysms should be clipped.
- Elderly patients (> 70 years) with either poor-grade aSAH (World Federation of Neurological Surgeons [WFNS] score of IV/V) or aneurysms of the basilar apex should be coiled.
- Patients who receive either intervention should have follow-up vascular imaging (time frame to be individualized) with strong consideration of retreatment if there is remnant growth.

- Anesthetic management during intervention should include minimization of intraoperative hypotension (mean arterial pressure [MAP] decrease > 50%) and hyperglycemia (glucose > 129 mg/dL)

Craniotomy With Clipping

- First performed in 1937; note that the first operative microscope was used in 1960, so the early neurosurgeons who performed aneurysm clippings did so without the benefit of the microscope.
- Involves opening the skull and manipulating brain tissue to access the aneurysm, increasing risk of complications associated with neurosurgery (i.e., infection and secondary injury).
- Higher rate of complete obliteration than coiling (81% vs. 58%)
- Lower rate of late rebleeding than coiling (0.9% vs. 2.9%)
- Higher rate of death and disability than coiling (31% vs. 24%)

Endovascular Coiling

- First performed in 1991; earlier techniques of balloon occlusion were done in the 1980s, but had very high complication rates.
- Involves large-artery access (usually femoral), with threading of the catheter up to the brain, similar to the process described in ischemic stroke mechanical intervention.
- Less invasive than craniotomy for clipping, but then only radiographic visibility of aneurysm
- Shorter recovery time and shorter length of stay than craniotomy approach
- Trend is toward more cases being appropriate for coiling due to improvements in technology, technique, and expertise of practitioners.

FAST FACTS in a NUTSHELL

Despite the advances in brain vascular imaging, up to 15% of patients are discharged from acute care with no documented cause of their SAH. In other words, no secondary prevention has been possible. They will have the usual risk factors controlled with the hope that that is enough to keep them from having another SAH. Causes of these SAHs with no angiographic evidence of aneurysm have been reported to be perforating arteries, venous hemorrhages, and intramural hematoma.

AVM OBLITERATION

Selection of intervention is based on the size and location of the AVM, as well as patient age and comorbid conditions, similar to aneurysm treatment decisions.

Surgical Removal

- Involves craniotomy approach and surgical excision of the lesion
- Indicated for medically stable patients, with small, uncomplicated lesions

Endovascular Embolization

- Involves a large-artery approach and use of particulate or embolizing agents
- Often utilized to stabilize or reduce the lesion size prior to surgery to reduce the incidence of intraoperative bleeding
- Most successful when combination therapy is used, and embolization is followed by surgery or radiation therapy

- Indicated for those patients for whom surgery or endo-vascular approach is not feasible
  - Examples are lesions in the thalamus, basal ganglia, and brainstem
- Involves use of gamma knife, linear accelerators, or proton beam radiation
- Often utilized after surgery or endovascular emboliza-tion to eliminate any remaining lesion
- Not indicated for large AVMs unless a staged approach using multiple treatments is possible

═══════════════════════════════════FAST FACTS in a NUTSHELL

Some individuals with a large AVM show signs of cog-nitive impairment as their presenting symptom. The changes are usually subtle, such as a change in person-ality or mild memory loss, but may progress to demen-tia. The decline is likely due to chronic diversion of blood from the cerebral tissue—an intracranial steal phenomenon.

CONTROL OF INTRACRANIAL PRESSURE

Surgical Excision of Hematoma

- Continues to be controversial, but general guidelines have been established with the following indications for surgery:
  - Patients with cerebellar hemorrhage who are deteriorating neurologically or have brainstem com-pression and/or hydrocephalus from ventricular obstruction
  - Patients with lobar clots greater than 30 mL that are within 1 cm of the surface
- Optimal time frame for surgery has not been standardized

Hemicraniectomy

- Removal of bone flap (see Chapter 10 for detailed discussion)
- Indication in hemorrhagic stroke remains controversial

External Ventricular Device, a.k.a. Ventriculostomy

- Catheter placed through burr hole in skull, and positioned in lateral ventricle
- Two purposes: (a) drainage of cerebral spinal fluid (CSF) to control intracranial pressure (ICP), and (b) monitoring of ICP values
- A third purpose is under investigation currently; that is, administration of tissue plasminogen activator (tPA) into the ventricle for patients with intraventricular hemorrhage (IVH).
  - The theoretical application is that the thrombolytic dissolves clots that form on the arachnoid villi that line the ventricles and drain the CSF.
  - Blood in the ventricles impedes CSF drainage, either through normal CSF channels or through the external ventricular device (EVD), leading to hydrocephalus.
- The permanent version is a ventriculo-peritoneal (VP) shunt.
  - Permanent CSF diversion from the ventricle to the peritoneal cavity via a tube
  - The purpose is long-term prevention of hydrocephalus that developed due to IVH and blockage of the normal CSF drainage pathway.

FAST FACTS in a NUTSHELL

Prevention of hydrocephalus through CSF diversion has been associated with a lower incidence of vasospasm, and thus provides secondary prevention of ischemic stroke. Vasospasm, if unresolved, can result in secondary ischemic stroke in the territory normally supplied by the spastic vessels.

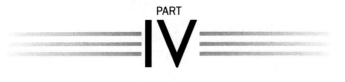

PART

IV

Key Elements of Stroke Care

12

Prehospital and Emergency Department

Prehospital care of the stroke patient is one of the areas that has seen the most change since 1996, the year that intravenous (IV) tissue plasminogen activator (tPA) was approved by the Food and Drug Administration (FDA). The level of response has been raised, requirements for stroke education have been established, protocols have been developed and amended, and specific parameters for measuring the quality of emergency medical services (EMS) care have been determined. The role of prehospital personnel is now recognized as the critical first step in the acute stroke care continuum. No longer does the EMS professional simply drop off the suspected stroke patient in the emergency department (ED), where the ED nurse starts at the beginning with assessment and vital sign documentation. Now EMS personnel take the patient directly to the computed tomography (CT) scanner, giving report to the ED nurse/provider en route; their documentation of last known well (LKW) time, neurologic assessment, medications, and family contact are recognized as important elements in the documentation of the continuum of care. The ED personnel are well trained to multitask, and an effective team is able

(continued)

> *(continued)*
>
> *to receive, identify, evaluate, treat, and obtain access to stroke expertise within a very short time frame. Just as their prehospital colleagues have parameters for measuring response times, so does the ED team.*

In this chapter, you will learn:

1. Recommendations for prehospital evaluation and management
2. Quality parameters for measuring prehospital response processes
3. Hyperacute blood pressure management guidelines
4. IV tPA considerations pre- and post-administration of drug
5. Dysphagia screening: rationale and tools
6. Role of telemedicine in acute stroke evaluation

PREHOSPITAL

Primary goals are rapid evaluation, early stabilization, neurologic evaluation, and rapid transport and triage to an appropriate stroke-capable hospital (Alberts et al., 2011). Key components of effective prehospital operation include:

- Brief, standardized neurologic assessment—Cincinnati Prehospital Scale, or Los Angeles Prehospital Scale
- Knowledge of the capabilities of the hospitals in their region; each stroke center should provide education and information about its capabilities to the EMS who bring them stroke patients
- List of certified stroke centers. This varies by state, but many states provide a list of certified stroke centers online
- Representatives of the area's EMS serve as members of the stroke center multidisciplinary stroke team
- Consideration for air medical transport is recommended if ground transport to the nearest stroke-capable hospital is more than 1 hour.

Specific recommendations are listed in the Guidelines for Early Management of Patients with Acute Ischemic Stroke, from the American Heart Association/American Stroke Association (Jauch et al., 2013).

- Also includes what is NOT recommended:
  - Intervention for hypertension—only if directed by medical command
  - Excess IV fluid
  - Dextrose-containing fluids in nonhypoglycemic patients
  - Oral medications
  - Any delay in transport for prehospital interventions
- Quality oversight: As with nursing, EMS has parameters for measuring quality of prehospital care (Acker et al., 2007)
  - Time between receipt of call and dispatch of the response team is less than 90 seconds.
  - EMS response time is less than 8 minutes (time elapsed from receipt of call by the dispatch entity to arrival on scene of a properly equipped and staffed ambulance).
  - Dispatch time less than 1 minute
  - Turnout time (time call received to the unit being en route) is less than 1 minute.
  - The on-scene time is les than 15 minutes (barring extenuating circumstances such as extrication difficulties).
  - Travel time is equivalent to trauma or acute myocardial infarction calls.

===================================*FAST FACTS in a NUTSHELL*

Many nurses do not understand the difference between an emergency medical technician (EMT) and a paramedic. There are significant differences: An EMT receives 120 to 150 hours of training, and cannot start IVs or give injections. A paramedic receives 1,200 to 1,800 hours of training, with many earning a 2-year degree; paramedics can start IVs and give injections. In many communities, the majority of the prehospital personnel are volunteers.

IN THE ED: STROKE-ALERT PROCESS

The Golden Hour

- Refers to the time from patient arrival until IV tPA is administered (Figure 12.1)
- Critical steps to be accomplished during that time were established by the National Institute of Neurological Disorders and Stroke (NINDS).
  - Process should be accomplished within 60 minutes for 80% or more of treated patients.

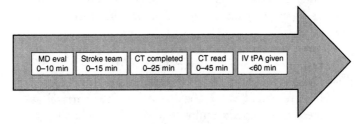

FIGURE 12.1 Golden Hour Components for stroke care.

FAST FACTS in a NUTSHELL

The Golden Hour was first described by R. Adams Cowley, MD, in the 1960s. From his observations in post-World War II Europe, and then in Baltimore, Dr. Cowley recognized that the sooner trauma patients reached definitive care—particularly if they arrived within 60 minutes of being injured—the better their chance of survival. The term has come to represent the critical first 60 minutes for many populations, with stroke being one of them.

Initial Evaluation

The primary goal is to identify patients with possible stroke as well as to exclude stroke mimics. These steps are often accomplished as a team effort, in the hallway or CT suite; in other words, the Golden Hour is not a linear process.

- Airway, breathing, circulation (ABCs)
- Patient history—confirm LKW time, review medical history, particularly related to eligibility for therapeutic interventions
- Neurologic assessment using a standardized tool such as National Institutes of Health Stroke Scale (NIHSS) or Canadian Neurological Scale
    - Standardized assessment tools can be performed rapidly and ensure consistency among health care providers
- Stroke team notification—With prenotification by EMS, the stroke team is often waiting at the ED when the patient arrives
    - Electrocardiogram (EKG) to assess for concurrent myocardial ischemia or arrhythmias
    - Oxygen saturation to assess for hypoxia
    - Blood tests—Ideally drawn by EMS shortly before arrival to ED; otherwise drawn as early as possible in the ED (see Chapter 6 for a list)
- In select patients, the following tests may also be done but should not delay intervention decision
    - Chest x-ray if lung disease suspected
    - Lumbar puncture if subarachnoid hemorrhage (SAH) is suspected and CT is negative for blood
    - Electroencephalogram (EEG) if seizures are suspected

Blood Pressure Management

Numerous published studies have failed to demonstrate a consensus on a specific systolic blood pressure (BP) or mean arterial pressure (MAP) for ischemic stroke, intracerebral hemorrhage (ICH), and SAH. Below are general recommendations from the respective guidelines, but all agree that individual patient condition and comorbidities will affect their optimal BP. See Chapter 13 for further discussion about BP management and cerebral autoregulation.

- Hemorrhagic stroke:
    - Upper limit for systolic BP: SAH = 160 mmHg; ICH = 150 to 220 mmHg

- Lower limit is based on patient's premorbid blood pressure and current condition. Care should be taken when administering an antihypertensive to not "overshoot" the goal, with resulting hypotension.
- Ischemic stroke:
  - Upper limit = 220/105 mmHg; antihypertensive medications should be given as ordered with close monitoring to determine whether goal was met, if there is need for more medication, or a need to address hypotension.
  - Lower limit is based on patient's premorbid blood pressure and current condition. Care should be taken when administering an antihypertensive to not "overshoot" the goal, with resulting hypotension. Swelling accompanies ischemic stroke and perfusion of the ischemic penumbra is dependent on adequate blood pressure.

Blood Sugar Management

- Recommendations vary as to specific target values for upper and lower limits.
- Glucose levels greater than 150 mg/dL should be treated whether the patient is diabetic or not; care should be taken that corrective measures do not induce hypoglycemia.
  - Especially important in patients who have received thrombolytics
  - Evidence indicates that sustained blood sugar levels greater than 200 during the first 24 hours are associated with worse outcomes. See Chapter 13 for further discussion of effects/management of glucose levels.

Temperature Management

- A temperature higher than 99.6°F or 37.5°C should be treated to achieve euthermia, as increased temperature is associated with worse outcomes. See Chapter 13 for discussion of effects/management of hyperthermia. Hypothermia as a therapeutic option will be addressed in Chapter 14.

Thrombolytic Administration

- Inclusion/exclusion criteria have been reviewed by the team
- Patient and/or family members have been informed of risk/benefits of tPA
  - For treatment within the 3-hour window, no written consent is necessary
  - For treatment within the 3- to 4.5-hour window, written consent is required
  - Consider using a fact sheet to augment the verbal discussion.
- BP is less than 185/110 mmHg
- Consider having a second nurse to assist during the initial hour of stroke alert.
  - Rapid acquisition and administration of antihypertensive if indicated
  - Second IV site established
  - Ensure rapid set-up, dose check, and administration of tPA (see Chapter 9 for tPA administration guidelines).
  - If a bladder catheter is indicated, it should be inserted prior to tPA administration, or held for a minimum of 30 minutes after infusion.
  - Nasogastric (NG) tubes are only indicated in the ED if there is nausea/vomiting and concern for aspiration risk.
- Frequent neurologic checks and vital sign documentation ensure early detection of any change in patient status; see Chapter 9 for the schedule.
- If bleeding is noted, or angioedema is evident, discontinue the infusion, notify the provider, and monitor the patient for anaphylaxis.

A patient presents to the ED with aphasia, right hemiparesis, and time from symptom onset of 1.5 hours. A stat CT of the head is done, which shows an infarct involving 40% of the left middle cerebral artery (MCA) territory, but no hemorrhage. Will you start to mix the tPA? No. CT findings involving more than one third of the MCA territory indicate a warning to providers that treatment with IV tPA may produce hemorrhagic conversion. So, even though tPA is a treatment for ischemic stroke, large infarcts are more risky.

Endovascular Intervention

A decision to proceed with endovascular intervention may be made following initiation of IV tPA or for patients ineligible for IV tPA.

- Review of CT, CTA, or MRA with evidence of thrombus in the proximal portion of one of the major cerebral arteries
- As with IV tPA, the earlier the treatment, the better the outcome.
- Written permission is required as this is an invasive procedure.
  - Having a fact sheet to augment the discussion with the patient and/or the family is very helpful.
- The nurse accompanies the patient to the intervention suite once the team is assembled and ready.
  - Varies with each organization as to whether this is an ED nurse or intensive care unit (ICU) nurse.
- Post endovascular intervention, the schedule for frequent neurologic checks and vital signs is restarted from the time of the end of the procedure whether IV tPA had been given or not.

- A nursing bedside dysphagia screen differs from full evaluation performed by a speech and language pathologist (SLP).
  - Reduces aspiration pneumonia incidence when performed prior to any oral intake and when measures are taken to maintain nothing by mouth (NPO) until a full evaluation can be performed by an SLP (Hinchey et al., 2005)
  - Numerous tools have been reported with varying results
    - Dysphagia screening was not endorsed by the National Quality Forum (NQF) due to lack of clinical trials identifying the optimal screening tool (Donovan et al., 2013). The NQF is a nonprofit organization that reviews, endorses, and recommends use of standardized health care performance measures. Their endorsements and recommendations are utilized by the federal government and many private-sector entities.
    - As a result, the dysphagia measure was removed from the Get With the Guidelines stroke guidelines and retired from The Joint Commission performance standards in 2012.
  - With pneumonia a common complication of stroke, all experts agree that screening for aspiration is important and *should* still be done to prevent aspiration and inadequate hydration/nutrition.
  - The American Speech-Language-Hearing Association (ASHA) supports the utilization of a nursing screening process.
  - Use of a water swallow trial has been found to be valid, but more research is needed regarding the implementation and interpretation of results. In the meantime, experts recommend that multidisciplinary teams continue to implement continuous quality improvement (CQI) processes to ensure optimal training for nurses

who perform the dysphagia screens and to review outcomes data in their organization (Donovan et al., 2013).
- For patients who cannot tolerate oral fluids, isotonic IV fluids such as Ringer's solution or normal (0.9%) saline should utilized for at least the first 24 hours.

Use of Telestroke (Telemedicine)

- The term "telestroke" was first used in the 1990s to describe interactive telemedicine in acute stroke evaluation and intervention.
- Recommended for increasing access to acute stroke care in underserved areas
  - A stroke-neurology expert can view and interact with the patient and the patient can view the care provider via two-way audio-video technology.
  - Provides expert consultation without "being there"
- Facilitates initiation of interventions proven to reduce complications and stroke recurrence
  - Proven to shorten door-to-needle time in patients receiving IV tPA
- Facilitates identification and transfer of patients for tertiary care interventions

FAST FACTS in a NUTSHELL

Telestroke technology not only facilitates rapid identification and treatment/transport, but it also facilitates identification of patients for whom transfer is not indicated. Examples are stable, small-territory ischemic strokes that can be managed by the community hospital, and devastating hemorrhagic strokes for which there is no acute intervention; comfort measures can be provided to these patients in the community hospital. Telestroke eliminates unnecessary, expensive transport, which has the benefit of controlling health care costs as well as saving the family from traveling a distance.

- Length of stay in the ED should be less than 3 hours (Jauch et al., 2013).
- Varies with each organization, but optimal hand-off between an ED nurse and an inpatient unit nurse is via face-to-face hand-off communication.
  - A neurologic assessment is done together to ensure agreement on current status.
  - Review of schedule for neurologic checks and vital signs for postintervention patients
  - Review of plan of care: goals for BP, temperature, blood sugar
  - Review of family contacts and patient belongings

13

In the Stroke Unit

It has long been established that patients who receive care in a specialized stroke unit, where the nurses and providers are educated and competent to provide the unique care required by stroke patients, have better outcomes: There is a 17% to 28% reduction in deaths, a 7% increase in being able to live at home, and an 8% reduction in lengths of stay (Langhorne et al., 1997). The exact structure of a stroke unit will be unique to each organization, but the basic concepts will be consistent: a defined group of beds, staff, equipment, and protocols that are used for the care of acute stroke patients. A stroke unit is not necessarily a geographically distinct hospital unit, but is an area with the capabilities noted above, and is the location where the majority of stroke patients are cared for in that facility. The stroke unit may or may not have intensive care units (ICUs) incorporated—many operate as step-down units. This chapter focuses on the care aspects of all stroke patients in the hospital—whether in the stroke unit or the ICU. Chapter 14 will cover the care aspects of stroke patients specific to the ICU.

In this chapter, you will learn:

1. Cerebral autoregulation: why blood pressure (BP) management is so critical
2. The rationale behind tight blood sugar and temperature management
3. Mobilization: safety versus therapeutics
4. The difference between functional assessment scores and severity scores

FAST FACTS in a NUTSHELL

Cerebral autoregulation is the ability of the brain to adjust to changes in systemic BP, ensuring steady cerebral perfusion despite extremes of systemic pressure. This is accomplished through a complex system of mechanisms acting to adjust the resistance of cerebral vascular beds. In an injured brain, these hemodynamics are impaired or abolished leaving the cerebral blood flow at the mercy of systemic perfusion pressure. Ischemic brain tissue has increased metabolic demand, and along with increased ICP due to edema, makes the case for the importance of close BP management—not too high and not too low.

BP MANAGEMENT

- BP management is one of the most important functions that a nurse caring for a stroke patient performs.
  - Nursing vigilance and response can impact the patient's ultimate functional recovery.
- If systemic BP rises too high, the blood–brain barrier may be disrupted, resulting in increasing cerebral edema, hemorrhagic transformation, or expansion of hemorrhagic stroke.
  - Patients with chronic hypertension and sustained hypertension are especially predisposed to these complications.

- For subarachnoid hemorrhage (SAH) patients, once an aneurysm is secure, an increase in BP is permitted; an upper limit of 200 mmHg is recommended (Connolly et al., 2012).
- If systemic BP is reduced dramatically, perfusion pressure may be inadequate for the penumbra, resulting in extension of the infarct, or loss of the penumbra.
  - Patients with chronic hypertension are especially susceptible and are at risk even at BPs that are "normal."
- A BP outside the specified parameters may not produce immediate clinical changes and the patient may look "fine," but has been shown to impact functional recovery down the road.
- Constipation should be avoided; a stool softener should be ordered to minimize straining, which can cause spikes in BP.
- Nursing considerations:
  - If an automatic cuff is utilized, high and low alarms should be set according to parameters ordered for that patient.
  - Parameters will vary according to the patient's history, and type and size of the stroke.

TEMPERATURE MANAGEMENT

- Brain temperature is warmer than core body temperature by almost a degree
- Hyperthermia increases metabolic demand on the already-injured brain; it also accelerates the ischemic cascade, thus contributing to the conversion of penumbra to infarct.
- Hyperthermia occurs in up to 54% of SAH patients.
- Hyperthermia within the first 24 hours has been associated with a twofold increase in short-term mortality.
- Nursing considerations:
  - Acetaminophen, aspirin, or ibuprofen should be administered as needed.
  - Blankets should be limited; room temperature should not be excessively warm
    - Education of family members is important so that they do not add blankets.

BLOOD SUGAR MANAGEMENT

- Hyperglycemia increases anaerobic metabolism, lactic acidosis, and free-radical production.
  - Hyperglycemia leads to infarct expansion, hemorrhagic transformation, and reduced recanalization with thrombolytics, associated with increased length of stay, and increased mortality.
- Once clinically stable, the goal for blood glucose is generally less than 140 mg/dL.
- Intravenous (IV) solutions containing glucose should not be used.
- Insulin drips are often utilized to ensure tight control.
- Nursing consideration: If a sliding-scale method is utilized, ensure that a schedule is followed and that treatment is punctual to avoid peaks and valleys.

VENOUS THROMBOEMBOLUS PREVENTION: ALSO REFERRED TO AS DEEP VEIN THROMBOSIS (DVT)

- Stroke patients spend more than 50% of their time in bed during the first 2 weeks.
- Immobility and limb paralysis make stroke patients especially susceptible to venous thromboembolus (VTE).
- Most effective prevention is early mobilization
- Minimize dependent edema with careful positioning of limbs.
- Unfractionated heparin, low-molecular-weight heparin, and heparinoids are effective but contraindicated for patients with hemorrhagic strokes or large territory ischemic strokes.
  - Once aneurysms are secure, SAH patients may receive heparin.
- Sequential compression devices (SCDs) have had mixed reviews but are recommended for patients who cannot receive pharmaceutical therapy.

- Nursing considerations: (a) SCDs work better when actually on the patient and power is turned on; (b) patients and families need education about the need for these devices so they do not take them off.
- Patients with pulmonary embolus from VTE in the lower extremity and a contraindication for antithrombotic treatment may benefit from placement of an inferior venal cava filter.

══════════════════════════════ *FAST FACTS in a NUTSHELL*

Thromboembolic deterrent (TED) stockings should not be used for the stroke population. They are difficult to put on, and are rarely put on by the patient who would know if they "felt right." Many stroke patients have sensory and/or communication deficit, or they may have an altered level of consciousness. So they either are not aware of a bad fit, or they cannot tell anyone. Results from the CLOTS-1 trial (Clots in Legs or Stockings After Stroke), reported in *Lancet* (2009), indicated that although graduated compression stockings were effective in surgical patients, they were not effective in stroke patients, and the potential for harm made them something to avoid.

CARDIAC MONITORING

- Patients with large deficits and right hemispheric strokes are at increased risk for myocardial infarction, heart failure, and atrial fibrillation.
- Patients with SAH are at risk for "stunned myocardium" with cardiac dysrhythmias (see Chapter 14 for a discussion).
- Cardiac monitoring for the first 24 hours is required; extended monitoring may be indicated.
- Recent studies have shown that 72-hour Holter monitoring may be more effective than 24-hour monitoring in identifying atrial fibrillation and other serious arrhythmias.

NUTRITION MANAGEMENT

- Dehydration and malnutrition may slow recovery; dehydration is a potential cause of VTE.
- Dysphagia screening is not just for the emergency department (ED)—any change in level of consciousness should prompt the nurse to rescreen the patient for swallow competence.
- Patients who cannot tolerate oral nutrition should receive IV fluid support of Ringer's solution or normal saline at a rate that ensures proper hydration (varies with each patient condition).
- If the patient fails the bedside nursing dysphagia screen, consultation with a speech and language pathologist (SLP) is indicated.
  - Video barium swallow may be ordered in which patient will swallow barium, or foods coated with barium, while fluoroscopic examination is done to assess swallow competence.
  - Consultation with a dietitian may also be indicated to determine calorie needs and appropriate nutritional support.
  - A nasogastric tube (NG) is often utilized short term for nutrition and medication administration.
  - A percutaneous endoscopic gastrostomy (PEG) tube may be indicated if long-term (more than 6–8 weeks) nutrition support is anticipated; most long-term care facilities do not accept patients with an NG tube.
- Nursing considerations:
  - Aggressive oral care will minimize the bacterial count in the mouth and decrease the risk of aspiration pneumonia.
  - The presence of an NG tube does not eliminate the risk of aspiration.
    - Routine monitoring of NG position and the amount of residual material in the stomach are key components of care.

- For patients who can tolerate oral intake, basic principles of feeding include:
  - Sitting in a high Fowler's position, preferably in a chair and remaining seated upright for 30 minutes after meals.
  - Recommendations of the SLP should be followed: Head positioning during swallow (chin tuck or neck extension) and thickening of fluids
  - Mouth care should be performed prior to feeding (facilitates sensation and production of saliva); mouth care should be performed after eating to observe whether the patient is pocketing food/remove food.
  - Pulmonary status should be assessed after eating (Pugh et al., 2012).

MOBILIZATION

- The rehabilitation team should be consulted early to develop a plan for rehabilitation.
- Passive range of motion can be implemented by nurses during the first 24 hours.
- Families can be instructed to perform range-of-motion exercises; this is an excellent opportunity to involve the family in the care of the patient.
- Nursing considerations:
  - When initially getting the patient out of bed (OOB), monitor BP sitting and standing: If a significant increase or decrease is noted, the patient should be returned to bed and the health care provider notified.
    - If autoregulation has been impacted, patient will be dependent on systemic pressure for perfusion; be aware of change in neurologic status while sitting OOB, as it may be a sign of decreased perfusion. If this is noted, patient should be returned to bed and monitored for return to previous neurologic status. If this does not occur, notify the health care provider.

- If the patient is ambulatory, note the presence of visual field defect, gaze palsy, or neglect that may impact ability to transfer in and out of bed or ambulate safely.
- For patients with significant upper extremity weakness:
  - Shoulder subluxation is a common and painful complication that can inhibit recovery.
  - Avoid pulling on affected arm and shoulder when getting OOB or when repositioning in bed.
  - Position arm on small pillow to minimize weight of limb pulling on shoulder joint, to minimize dependent edema, and to prevent limb slipping off the side of the bed and possibly getting caught between the side rail and mattress.
- For patients with significant lower extremity weakness:
  - Position the leg on a small pillow to minimize dependent edema and to prevent external rotation of the hip

FAST FACTS in a NUTSHELL

It is the responsibility of the entire health care team to ensure mobilization for stroke patients, whether it be via range-of-motion exercises in bed or assisted ambulation. Physical therapists do mobilization as part of therapy; it is the neuroscience nurse's role to facilitate and augment that therapy when getting the patient up to the chair or the bathroom. Nurses on a stroke unit should be competent in proper body mechanics and techniques for facilitating safe mobility for patients with deficits.

SAFETY MEASURES

- Falls precautions
  - Motor, sensory, communication, visual, balance, and cognitive deficits put stroke patients at increased risk for falls.

- Nursing considerations:
  - Frequent nursing rounds have demonstrated reduced fall rates.
  - Frequent orientation and reiteration of instructions is necessary.
  - Call bells should be within reach and located on the patient's unaffected side.
  - Bedside tables should be placed on the patient's unaffected side
  - Offer toileting at least every 2 hours while awake, and every 4 hours at night.
- Skin precautions
  - Skin breakdown occurs in 9% of all hospitalized patients.
  - Stroke patients are at increased risk due to immobility, loss of sensation, incontinence, and impaired circulation; in addition, diabetes is a common comorbid condition that increases the risk of skin breakdown.
  - Nursing considerations:
    - An assessment tool to evaluate and predict risk should be utilized.
    - Patients should be repositioned every 2 hours using proper techniques to avoid excessive friction; skin assessment should be done with each repositioning.
    - Skin should be kept clean and dry.

═══════════════════════════════*FAST FACTS in a NUTSHELL*

Infections are common following stroke and adversely influence the outcome. Research evidence indicates that stroke leads to suppression of immune responses, which predisposes to infection. Poststroke immunodepression has been associated with increased susceptibility to infection—the most common being urinary tract infection (UTI) and pneumonia.

- Infection prevention
  - Pneumonia is responsible for approximately 35% of acute stroke patient deaths.
    - Pneumonia incidence is highest with mechanical ventilation, dysphagia, and prolonged immobility, which leads to atelectasis.
  - UTIs occur in up to 60% of stroke patients, and are associated with poor outcomes.
    - Incidence of UTIs is highest with indwelling catheter placement.
    - Loss of sphincter control increases the risk for UTI.
  - Nursing considerations:
    - Early mobilization and frequent repositioning are critical.
    - Dysphagia screening protocols should be implemented, as discussed in Chapter 12.
    - Regular, thorough pulmonary hygiene should be performed.
    - Avoidance of indwelling catheters is important; if one is necessary, meticulous catheter care and removal as soon as possible will minimize risk.
    - Frequent hand washing—both nurse and patient—will minimize risk.
    - Education and reassurance for the patient regarding the need for an endotracheal tube and/or bladder catheter, and the need for not pulling/touching these tubes, will reduce anxiety and minimize risk.

FUNCTIONAL ASSESSMENT

- Ideally, a functional assessment is done at admission, basing the score on pre-event status, and at discharge from acute care; it is also done at strategic points along the recovery continuum.

- The purpose of the preadmission status score is to provide a functional baseline for discharge planning.
- The purpose of the discharge score is to establish functional status.
  - Calculation of change from prehospital score indicates the effect of stroke.
  - Population scores (mean, median, range) are representative of each stroke-type outcome.
- The Barthel Index (BI) measures the patient's performance in 10 activities of daily living (ADLs).
  - Developed in 1965 (Mahoney & Barthel, 1965)
  - Categories are feeding, bathing, grooming, dressing, bowels, bladder, toilet use, transfers, mobility, and stairs.
    - Each is scored as 0, 5, or 10 with 0 = dependent, and 10 = independent.
  - Total score range is 0 (totally dependent) to 100 (fully independent).
    - Score of more than 60 is considered to be compatible with good outcomes/ability to live at home.
- Modified Rankin Scale (mRS) measures independence rather than performance of specific tasks.
  - Developed in 1957 (Rankin, 1957) and modified to its current format in 1988 (Beaglehole, 1988)
  - Score range is 0 (fully independent) to 6 (dead), with 5 (severely disabled, totally dependent) being the highest possible score for patients being discharged alive.
    - Score of 4: Moderately severe disability, unable to walk without assistance, and unable to attend to ADLs without assistance.
    - Score of 3: Moderate disability, but able to walk without assistance.
    - Score of 0 to 2: Considered to be compatible with good outcomes.

Functional scores (mRS and BI) differ from severity scores (NIHSS, Hunt & Hess, Fisher, ICH, and mICH) in that they have been demonstrated to provide a measure of functional ability, or independence, whereas the severity scores are utilized to determine not only the amount of deficit, but also the risk for mortality. The NIHSS is unique in that it has been utilized as both a severity score and a functional score. The Modified ICH Score takes into account comorbid conditions that increase the risk for mortality over and above the size and location of the bleed.

14

In the Intensive Care Unit

Susan J. Pazuchanics

Neuroscience nursing in the intensive care unit (ICU) is focused on an astute neurologic assessment of the patient. The ability to identify subtle changes in a patient's condition can have a significant impact on patient outcome . . . as we know, "time is brain." Frequent bedside assessments are often supplemented with advanced neurologic monitoring and testing capabilities. Neuroscience nurses in the ICU are detectives piecing together a puzzle, relying on accurate assessments and monitored values, to identify changes that may negatively impact the patient. Neurologic changes can be quite subtle, and neuroscience ICU nurses must be particularly adept at utilizing that "gut feeling" that has been ascribed to nurses in general. When one considers the exciting developments in neuroscience as a whole, and especially within stroke care, neuroscience nursing represents the new frontier in nursing. Neuroscience nursing demands that the nurses be knowledgeable, competent, keenly observant, and responsive to subtle changes.

In this chapter, you will learn:

1. Hemorrhagic and ischemic stroke care in the ICU
2. Management of increased intracranial pressure (ICP)

Treatment of increased ICP is based on the Monroe–Kellie Doctrine. The skull is a closed box that contains roughly 80% brain matter, 10% blood, and 10% cerebrospinal fluid (CSF). If one of the contents increases, then one of the other two must decrease. Treatment decisions are based on what item in the box can be altered to lower the pressure in the cranial vault.

ASSESSMENT

- In the ICU, neurological assessments include all the parts of the exam covered in Chapter 7, but on a more frequent schedule
- Cranial nerve assessment should be included in ICU nurses' neurological assessments (see Chapter 7)
  - In particular, patients with a posterior fossa stroke are especially at risk due to close proximity to the brainstem, which is where the majority of the cranial nerves originate
- Bedside handoff is essential
  - At shift transition, nursing personnel complete a joint neurologic exam so each provider can establish an agreed-on status for that patient.
  - The neurological exam affords providers a baseline assessment so subtle changes can be identified.
- Intensive neurologic monitoring may be used to assess for signs of deterioration related to conditions such as increasing cerebral edema or reperfusion syndrome.
- Continuous electrocardiogram (EKG) monitoring, along with frequent vital signs and nursing assessments, are routine expectations.
- Level of consciousness (LOC) is the first indicator of a neurologic change.
  - Variations in assessment should be reported to providers immediately.

POSTSTROKE COMPLICATIONS

Hemorrhagic Stroke Patients

- Seizures
  - About 20% to 25% of subarachnoid hemorrhage (SAH) patients will have seizures; most commonly after middle cerebral artery (MCA) rupture.
  - Blood on parenchymal tissue or an increased ICP can cause seizures.
  - Antiepileptics are often prescribed in the acute phase.
  - Nursing considerations:
    - Assess for other causes of seizures, such as electrolyte disturbances or ethanol withdrawal.
    - Prevent injury due to change in LOC: Pad side rails and institute safety measures, such as a low bed, and institute falls precautions.
    - Protect airway: supplemental oxygen, functioning-wall suction, and an oral suction tube should be readily available in the patient's room.
    - Continuous bedside electroencehalogram (EEG) monitoring may be required.
- Hydrocephalus
  - Usually presents in the first 24 hours after injury
  - Watch for a change in LOC.
  - A ventricular catheter may be placed to drain CSF; catheter care and nursing considerations are discussed later in this chapter.
- Rebleeding
  - Symptoms of rebleeding are related to an increase in intracranial pressure.
  - Intravenous vasoactive medications are used to decrease blood pressure or maintain hemodynamic parameters to limit risk of rebleeding or poor cerebral perfusion.
- Vasospasm
  - Common cause of neurologic deterioration after an SAH patient is initially stabilized
  - Usually occurs between days 4 and 10 following the original bleed
    - Can been seen up to 21 days post-SAH

- Transcranial Doppler (TCD) is useful in monitoring for vasospasm.
  - Ultrasound technology that monitors blood flow via the temporal window
- Treatment options
  - Triple H therapy: Hypertension, hemodilution, and hypervolemia
  - Vasoactive medications to keep a patient's blood pressure up
  - Isotonic fluids and/or albumin to establish hypervolemia and decrease blood viscosity
  - Magnesium and/or calcium channel blockers—vascular smooth muscle relaxants to decrease vasospasm
- Nursing considerations:
  - Look for sensory depression or drowsiness.
  - EKG changes frequently occur after SAH; while most abnormalities are benign, cardiac ischemia should be ruled out before assuming the change is of neurologic origin.
  - Cardiac markers and serial 12-lead EKGs may be warranted.

====FAST FACTS in a NUTSHELL

Patients with SAH often have cerebral salt wasting (CSW). Clinical symptoms of CSW include hyponatremia and polyuria. The low sodium state in CSW is caused by excessive removal of salt by the kidneys and is not a dilutional low sodium level as seen in syndrome of inappropriate antidiuretic hormone secretion (SIADH). Health care providers must be cognizant of the reasoning behind presenting symptoms and treat CSW with oral sodium replacement and/or hypertonic saline rather than fluid restriction, which would be detrimental to the SAH patient's outcome.

- Cerebral edema
  - Seen especially in the large middle cerebral artery stroke; leads to a steady decline in neurologic status
  - Mannitol and hypertonic saline decrease cerebral edema
  - Temperature management is also important and is discussed later in this chapter.
  - Nursing considerations:
    - Close neurological monitoring is essential; LOC changes are early signs.
    - Dextrose should be avoided in the majority of neuroscience patients.
  - As the body uses up the glucose content in the fluid, the water that remains crosses the blood–brain barrier and increases cerebral edema.
    - Isotonic fluids (0.9% normal saline or lactated Ringer's) are preferred.
- Hemorrhagic conversion
  - The natural hemorrhagic conversion rate has been reported to be between 0.6% and 10%.
  - In the National Institute of Neurological Diseases and Stroke (NINDS) trial, patients who received intravenous (IV) tissue plasminogen activator (tPA) had a 6.4% rate of hemorrhagic conversion.
  - Many are not clinically significant (clinical significance includes whether the patient is symptomatic, requiring change in treatment, or resulting in disability or death).
  - Petechial versus parenchymal hemorrhage
    - Petechial hemorrhage: Patchy hemorrhage often found on routine 24-hour imaging; patients usually asymptomatic
    - Parenchymal hemorrhage: Hemorrhage with mass effect; patient usually symptomatic
  - Blood pressure is a significant factor, especially in the first 24 hours after IV tPA.

– Elevation in blood pressure usually peaks 6 hours after tPA administration.
– For every 10 mmHg elevation in blood pressure after tPA is given, the odds of hemorrhage increase 59% (Butcher et al., 2010).
– Vasoactive medications may be administered as continuous infusions as needed if antihypertensive dosing is not effective.

POSTINTERVENTIONAL PROCEDURE PATIENT MANAGEMENT

- Vital signs and neurologic assessment (same as for IV tPA):
  - Every 15 minutes for 2 hours (starting at completion of procedure), then
  - Every 30 minutes for 6 hours, then
  - Every hour for 16 hours, then according to level of care
- Visualization of the groin puncture site and vascular checks of the distal pulses in the extremity used for the procedure
  - Every 15 minutes for the immediate 2 hours post-procedure, then every 30 minutes for 2 hours, then hourly
- Nursing considerations:
  - Assess the patient, groin site, and sheath leg for the following signs:
    – Hematoma development at the groin site
    – Swelling or bleeding at the sheath site
    – Development of a pseudoaneurysm, dissection of the artery, or clot formation
      • Complaint of increasing back or thigh pain
      • Pallor, pain, and paresthesia in the sheath extremity
    – Hemodynamic instability; that is, hypotension and tachycardia related to blood loss
    – Pulses: Dorsalis pedis and posterior tibial
    – A quick assessment technique is to place the pulse-oximetry probe on the toe of the sheath extremity

to monitor limb blood flow to identify complications early.

- Sheath management is similar to that of an arterial line, with a continuous pressure bag in place and the pressure line connected to the hemodynamic monitor with alarm limits on.

All stroke patients in intensive care are monitored for the development of increased ICP. Methods for decreasing ICP:

- Decrease stimulation to the patient
  - Limit visitors/physical stimulation
  - Do not cluster nursing care
  - Low lighting, limit white noise
  - Suction only when necessary
- Properly position patient
  - Head of the bed at 30 degrees unless contraindicated
  - Neck midline to allow venous drainage
  - No hip flexion; this will increase ICP
  - Remove all external irritants (i.e., wrinkled sheets, etc.)
- Monitor elimination and nutrition
  - Stool softeners daily; prevent urinary distension
  - Once the patient passes the swallowing screen, feeding should begin as soon as possible.
    - Patients who fail a swallow screen must have a speech therapy consult before oral intake is initiated.

FAST FACTS in a NUTSHELL

Cerebral reperfusion injury may occur in stroke patients following an intervention procedure. Cerebral reperfusion is defined as a deterioration of ischemic, but salvageable, brain tissue after reperfusion. Leukocytes and platelets play a part in this condition, which may lead to a fatal cerebral edema, intracranial hemorrhage (ICH), or an increase in the size of the initial stroke. A breakdown of the blood–brain barrier as a result of reperfusion injury may lead to vasogenic edema.

- Nursing considerations:
  - Enteral nutrition is often required in the care of stroke patients due to dysphagia.
  - Early nutrition is critical to:
    - Avoid transmigration of gut flora, which may lead to sepsis
    - Avoid third-spacing of intravascular fluids by maintaining nutritional balance and protein levels
  - Nasogastric tube or percutaneous endoscopic gastrostomy (PEG) tube may be placed to provide nutrition.
    - Tube placement should be confirmed with an x-ray prior to use.
- Administer sedation as ordered
  - Intravenous pain medications, sedatives, and/or paralytics may be utilized.
    - Ensure that pain and agitation control are provided consistently.
  - Medication-induced coma may be used to treat intractable intracranial hypertension.
    - Need to have a continuous EEG to monitor brainwave activity
    - Caution with kidney and liver failure patients due to drug metabolism and excretion
- Manage blood pressure
  - Mean arterial pressure (MAP) = [(2 × diastolic) + systolic]/3
    - In a normal brain, a MAP of about 60 is necessary to perfuse coronary arteries, brain, kidneys, but may not be adequate to perfuse an injured brain.
    - Patient-specific blood pressure goals should be strictly followed.
  - MAP – ICP = Cerebral perfusion pressure (CPP)
    - CPP should be 60 mmHg or higher unless contraindicated
  - See Chapter 13 for discussion of systemic blood pressure (BP) management and cerebral autoregulation.

- Nursing considerations:
  - Alarm limits in bedside monitoring equipment are set to patient-specific goals.
  - Consider other causes for increased BP:
    - Agitation—could be caused by fear, confusion, overstimulation, anger, feeling cold/hot/pain
    - Pain—bladder catheter, IV site, A-line, external-ventricular drain (EVD), surgical site, puncture site
  - BP parameters outside the ordered goals should be reassessed before action is taken—do not treat an isolated BP.
  - If antihypertensives are administered, BP is reassessed in 15 to 30 minutes to determine whether BP goals are being reached in a timely manner.
- Maintain fluid status and electrolyte balance
  - Normal saline solution is used for routine continuous IV fluid.
  - Hypertonic saline (> 0.9%) as a continuous infusion may be administered to replace low sodium levels.
  - Glucose levels—monitor every 6 hours or more often based on patient status.
  - Nursing considerations:
    - Frequent lab draws to monitor electrolyte levels when using hypertonic fluid replacement
    - Caution when correcting sodium levels to avoid causing central pontine myelinosis—watch for reduced level of consciousness, confusion, spasticity
    - Daily weights are useful to monitor patient fluid balance
- Administer diuretics for cerebral edema
  - Mannitol (osmotic diuretic) and hypertonic saline decrease ICP by pulling fluid out of the cerebral cell and back into the intravascular space.
  - 23.4% hypertonic saline IV boluses decrease severe cerebral edema
  - Nursing considerations:
    - Monitor electrolytes and serum osmolality during osmotic diuretic therapy.
    - Monitor for signs and symptoms of dehydration
    - Daily weights to monitor fluid balance

- Administer prophylactic antiepileptics
  - Nursing considerations:
    - Watch for decreased LOC.
- Drain CSF and monitor ICP
  - An EVD, or ventriculostomy, is commonly used to drain CSF, which can lower ICP.
    - Inserted into the nondominant ventricle via a burr hole
    - Considered to be the most accurate way to measure ICP (Morganstern et al., 2010)
  - Nursing considerations:
    - Catheters are gravity-based systems; drain height (in relation to the patient's position) is critical to the amount of CSF that will drain.
      - Catheter must be zeroed for an accurate ICP reading
        - Changes in patient position require releveling
      - The zero or releveling point for the catheter is usually the tragus or external auditory canal; the zero point is based on the provider orders.
      - Alarms should be set to patient-specific parameters.
    - Strict aseptic technique is essential to limit risk of hospital-acquired central nervous system (CNS) infection.
      - Prior to insertion, hair is clipped rather than shaved to decrease infection risk and allow for proper dressing adherence.
      - A mask and sterile gloves are worn.
      - Dressings must remain dry and intact.
    - Other devices to monitor ICP:
      - Subarachnoid bolt inserted via a burr hole
      - Epidural catheter inserted via a small drill hole
      - Intraparenchymal pressure monitor inserted via a cranial access bolt
- Control respiratory components
  - Cerebral oxygenation monitoring facilitates assessment of brain tissue perfusion and oxygenation.

- SjvO$_2$ catheter—Jugular venous oximetry measures jugular venous oxygen saturation
- Hyperventilation is avoided as hypocapnia is a potent vasoconstrictor.
- Hypercapnia is avoided as it is a potent vasodilator.
- Nursing considerations:
  - Diligent oral care decreases the risk of ventilator-associated pneumonia (VAP).
  - Epiglottis-level suctioning prevents oral flora from contaminating the lungs.
  - Head of bed at 30 degrees is effective in the prevention of VAP
- Institute normothermia or therapeutic hypothermia
  - Core body temperature goal is less than 37° C
  - Hypothermia (temperature at 33 to 35°C) for several days is used to reduce ICP when unable to be controlled with other measures
    - Hypothermia lowers cerebral cell metabolism, decreasing ICP.
  - Shivering is common, but increases metabolic demand and increases ICP.
    - Medications like Demerol, magnesium, and buspirone are beneficial in controlling shivering.
    - Nursing considerations:
      - Administer antipyretics as ordered to prevent fever.
      - During induction of hypothermia, monitor electrolytes and EKG for bradyarrhythmias.
      - Counterwarming is used to decrease shivering.
      - Hand warmers and surface warming are provided to decrease shivering without raising the patient's body temperature.
    - Skin care every 2 to 4 hours is a priority to monitor for breakdown or frostbite.
    - Rewarming phase must be done slowly to avoid rebound increases in ICP due to cerebral edema.
      - Electrolytes are monitored throughout the rewarming phase.
      - Potassium is replaced cautiously due to electrolyte shifts at the cellular level.

During hypothermia treatment, if the patient is not maintaining the set treatment goal temperature or the cooling machine is working harder to maintain the goal, consider infection or micro shivering as possible causes.

- Care post hemicraniectomy
  - Partial bone flap removal allows the size of the cranial vault to be altered, providing the brain room to swell, decreasing the threat of herniation.
  - Often seen in malignant MCA strokes with a large ischemic area
  - Nursing considerations:
    - Ensure use of a protective helmet when out of bed because the skull is no longer intact.
    - Optimal wound care is essential to limit skin flora exposure to the surgical site.
    - If the bone flap is stored in subcutaneous tissue (abdomen or thigh), provide wound care and monitor for signs of infection.
    - The bone flap (either the patient's own bone or prosthetic material) may be replaced in 6 to 8 weeks after the risk for swelling and increased ICP have passed.

15

Patient and Family as Members of the Team and Transitions From Acute Care

Multidisciplinary team members caring for acute stroke patients include physicians, bedside nurses, therapists, pharmacists, social workers, case managers, chaplains—and the patient and family members. The professional members of the team have well-defined roles, but the challenge with patients and families is that they are all different, with different skill and knowledge sets. Many health care professionals can attest to the fact that involving the patient and family in the plan of care from day one is vital in ensuring that a full team approach is possible, and that the best discharge plan can be established. As with all team dynamics, there should be a coordinator to ensure synchrony. Regardless of where the patient is cared for, one standard in stroke care is constant: It is the nurse who coordinates the various activities of the multidisciplinary team. The use of clinical pathways, standard orders, and protocols facilitate this process and can improve the quality of care and patient outcomes. Ultimately the neuroscience nurse has the opportunity and responsibility to advocate for the best care for his or her patients, and collaboration with the family members and caregivers will ensure that success.

In this chapter, you will learn:

1. Prioritization and timing of educational content
2. Potential pitfalls in family interaction
3. Discharge-planning criteria

FAST FACTS in a NUTSHELL

Therapeutic environment refers to the surrounding conditions in which factors like diseases impact the processes of care. The term has been utilized in many different care locations. In the acute care setting, therapeutic environment has been associated with medication and treatment, patient satisfaction, and psychosocial interaction. The effects of stroke in the acute care setting are threatening to both the patient and the family as they contemplate what the future might be like. Therefore, a therapeutic environment is especially important to minimize stress and ensure that the family members are engaged in the plan of care.

PATIENT AND FAMILY EDUCATION

- Patient and family readiness for education is unique to each case.
  - Pay attention—what problems/concerns has your patient or the family identified?
    - May be verbal or nonverbal expression (body language, mood)
  - Start with what they want to know—this allays anxiety and makes them more likely to pay attention to your message.
- Keep messages brief, focused, and simple.
  - Adult learners who have not had a stroke retain only about 30% of what they see and hear.
  - Ask them to tell you what they just heard—known as the teach-back method (Xu, 2012).

- Medications: "Let's review what each of these medications is for."
- Risk factors: "Let's review some strategies for controlling your diabetes."
- Signs and symptoms: "Can you tell me some symptoms of stroke other than the ones you experienced? What would you do if you experienced any of these symptoms?

■ Provide written material to reinforce content.
■ Briefly review what was presented the day before; if the information was not retained, repeat it.

- Prioritization of educational content
  ■ Monitoring equipment
  ■ Diagnostic tests and procedures—what they are and rationale for them
  ■ Medications
  ■ Plan of care, including anticipated length of stay
  ■ Type of stroke or transient ischemic attack (TIA)
  ■ Patient-specific risk factors
  ■ Importance of calling 911
  ■ Discharge medications and follow-up appointments
  ■ Contact information for questions/concerns after discharge
  ■ In-depth discussion about lifestyle factors that caused this stroke should be addressed in follow-up appointments.
    - Patients can be devastated as they adjust to the effects of the stroke and are then reminded that they did this to themselves.
    - Some patients may ask and demonstrate readiness to hear this, but care should be taken not to sound punitive.
  ■ Remember that these patients are usually anxious, overstimulated, sleep deprived, and may have cognitive impairment as result of the stroke . . . and their family members are not much different.
    - It will be the rare patient/family who can benefit from a detailed session of anatomy and pathophysiology.

- With respect for the patient/family—and the nurse's—time, educational content should be limited to "need to know."
- Resources for educational and support materials
  - American Stroke Association (ASA) and American Heart Association (AHA)
    - www.strokeassociation.org and www.americanheart.org
    - *Stroke Connection* magazine
    - Customizable patient education materials
  - National Stroke Association (NSA)
    - www.stroke.org
    - *Stroke Smart* magazine
  - Brain Attack Coalition
    - www.stroke-site.org
  - National Institutes of Neurological Diseases and Stroke (NINDS)
    - www.ninds.nih.org
  - Family Caregiver Alliance
    - www.caregiver.org
  - National Aphasia Association
    - www.aphasia.org

POTENTIAL PITFALLS IN PATIENT/FAMILY INTERACTIONS

- "Problem" patients or families
  - Remember that stroke represents an enormous threat to family structure and function.
    - Frequent reassurance and updates are very helpful
    - Utilize the active listening technique
    - Anticipate and stay ahead of their questions
    - Anger and frustration are likely not directed at you personally
    - Offer spiritual support
  - Multiple family members asking the same question
    - A designee should be established to avoid repetition as well as contradictory interpretation.

- One family member asking the same question to several different members of the team
  - Probably due to anxiety; speak with that family member about why he or she feels the need to keep asking the same question
- Lack of consensus on plan of care
  - Due to mixed messages from different members of the care team?
    - Reassure patient/family that you will clarify the discrepancies and communicate with all members of the care team.
  - Nurse presence when each provider sees the patient is essential
    - Ensure that each provider is aware of/agrees with the plan of care.
    - Communicate the plan to all members of team, including the patient and family.
  - Due to family dynamics?
    - Patient/family/care team meetings to ensure all hear the same message at the same time
  - Use the entire team, including spiritual support and patient advocates.

FAST FACTS in a NUTSHELL

All patients want to go home from the hospital and their family members want them home as well. Studies have shown that home health care results in improved functional outcomes and is more cost-effective than other discharge facilities. However, with three quarters of stroke survivors requiring care of family members in the home, the burden on family members can be overwhelming; it is the leading cause of institutionalization of stroke survivors. Careful discharge planning by the entire team involves not just assessing the patient's needs, but also evaluating the family's readiness and ability to provide ongoing support.

TRANSITION FROM ACUTE CARE

The patient's discharge disposition will be determined by the team based on:

	Home/ Home Care	Acute Rehabilitation	Skilled Nursing Facility
Ability to perform activities of daily living (ADLs)	Either independently or with assistance; appropriate person available in home	Has potential for return to independence with or without assistance	Limited potential for independence, or anticipation that it will take months to achieve
Ability to participate in therapy activities	Either with outpatient therapist and on his or her own	Tolerates minimum of 3 hours/day of combined therapies	Able to interact, but requires slower pace; or custodial care only
Other considerations	For home care services, must be homebound; with few exceptions, services approved as 60-day episodes	Must have medical comorbid conditions that require 24-hour care by health care professional	Must require daily skilled nursing or rehabilitation services that are only provided in an inpatient setting

- Long-term acute care hospital is a discharge option for a short-term acute care hospital if the patient will require long-term support in the form of ventilator management, pneumonia or sepsis management, seizure management, or other comorbid conditions that preclude a level of care other than acute care.
- Hospice care is a discharge option for patients for whom palliative care, or comfort care, has been selected.
  - Care can be delivered in a hospital, skilled nursing facility, inpatient hospice facility, or the home.

The greatest concern reported by caregivers was the transition from institutional setting to home; that is, processes for how to initiate/continue rehabilitation in the home setting. Stroke associations, support groups, help in the home, and therapy and counseling options were identified as important topics to address prior to transition to home.

FAMILY READINESS

- Assessment of family/caregivers needs and concerns is essential to help determine readiness for discharge plan.
  - Assessment tools are available for use throughout the care continuum (Miller et al., 2010).
- Prior to discharge, family/caregivers require knowledge about the extent and rationale of specific limitations, needs, or schedules so that they can either support the plan of care or realize that they cannot support it.
  - Positioning and handling, transfers and shoulder care, feeding precautions, communication strategies, and guidelines on promoting independence (not doing too much)
  - Comfort level with providing ADL support such as toileting, bathing, and dressing
  - Administration of medications like subcutaneous anticoagulants or insulin
  - Administration of tube feedings
  - Blood sugar testing
  - Need for transportation to doctor appointments and therapy appointments
- Symptoms of recurrent or new stroke and importance of calling 911

- Home environment evaluation by therapist to determine accessibility, safety, equipment needs, or need for modifications
- Information about community resources available for support
  - Provide detailed contact information—names, phone numbers, addresses, e-mail addresses

FAST FACTS in a NUTSHELL

Caregivers' advice to fellow stroke caregivers was gathered in a study published in 2002 by Bakas et al. The following recommendations were provided: (a) getting more information before discharge, (b) attending classes and support groups, (c) finding books or written materials about stroke, (d) keeping a running list of questions to ask, and (e) attending and participating in therapy sessions to learn what the survivors can do.

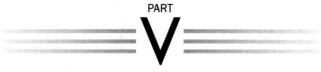

PART

V

Post–Acute Care Essentials

16

Rehabilitative Care

During the past decade, there has been a marked increase in knowledge regarding the potential of the brain to reorganize in response to both internal and external demands. There have been tremendous developments and changes in therapeutic and rehabilitative approaches to optimize functional recovery. In conjunction with improved acute care, these changes have resulted in improved functional recovery for cognitive deficits, motor deficits, as well as sensory and perceptual deficits.

Comprehensive stroke rehabilitation should include (a) Strategies for improvement of neurological, psychological, and cognitive deficits; (b) Strategies to assist with activities of daily living; (c) Prevention of secondary complications; (d) Strategies to optimize independence in the home environment; (e) Vocational therapies to maximize potential for return to work and for reintegration into society.

In this chapter, you will learn:

1. Common post-acute stroke complications
2. Specialized rehabilitation treatments and devices
3. Emerging strategies and research in stroke rehabilitation

THE BED IS NOT THE BATTLEGROUND

Whether the care setting post stroke is an inpatient rehabilitation center, a skilled nursing facility, or home with outpatient services, the multidisciplinary team should continue to function cohesively to ensure that the patient's needs are met. Nurses generally have the most direct contact with stroke patients and their caregivers, so they are often the coordinators of the care. In this capacity, nurses must be knowledgeable about the variety of services provided by the other members of the care team. Communication with the patient and family/caregiver, as well as the therapists, dieticians, pharmacists, and physicians is the key to synchronizing the complex needs of the stroke patient. Sometimes the needs overlap; for instance, cognitive deficits may need to be addressed by speech and language pathologists (SLPs), occupational therapists (OTs), and neuropsychologists. Therefore, the ideal situation is one in which all members of the care team collaborate with little concern for whose job it is, or who is coordinating the team.

POST-ACUTE COMPLICATIONS

- Shoulder pain
  - Occurs in up to 80% of stroke patients with upper extremity paresis and is result of traction on the arm during transfers and repositioning, or subluxation due to weight of paretic arm and poor positioning or support of the limb
  - Treatment involves progressive range-of-motion exercises, electrical stimulation, heat, anti-inflammatory agents, and analgesics.
  - Nursing considerations:
    - Ensure proper handling during transfers, ambulation, and repositioning in bed.

- Provide careful positioning of the affected limb at rest—either in a chair or in bed.
- Incontinence and constipation
  - Urinary and fecal incontinence are common, but usually resolve within 2 to 4 weeks.
  - Neurogenic bladder causes either urge incontinence or overflow incontinence, but is more common in patients with cognitive impairment.
  - May be due to urinary tract infection
  - Constipation becomes more common after first 2 weeks.
    - Inactivity, decreased fluid intake, and depression are causes.
  - Nursing considerations:
    - Establish a timed voiding program.
    - Establish a bowel training program.
    - Encourage activity to facilitate bowel motility.
    - Ensure adequate fluid intake and diet high in fiber.
    - Stool softeners and laxatives may be needed, at least temporarily.
- Depression
  - Common after stroke, with incidence of up to 80% reported
  - Due to psychological impact of loss of function/independence or due to biological impact of alteration of brain neurotransmitter function
  - Treatment involves antidepressants and psychotherapy
  - Nursing considerations:
    - Notify provider if the following are noted: apathy, crying or overt sadness, constant fatigue, sleep disturbance, appetite change, or suicidal thoughts
    - A variety of screening tools are available for use and have been helpful in identifying early signs of depression (Miller et al., 2010).

FAST FACTS in a NUTSHELL

Evidence has shown that patients treated with antidepressants even without depressive symptoms had better functional recovery. For several years, many providers started all their stroke patients on antidepressants during the acute hospital stay to ensure adequate blood level during the early rehabilitation phase. However, the side effects and drug interactions with these medications have led to recommendations that treatment be instituted only when symptoms are noted.

- Posttraumatic stress disorder (PTSD)
  - Recent studies have reported that 23% of stroke patients suffer PTSD within the first year and 11% experience chronic PTSD (defined as duration of longer than 3 months; Edmondson et al., 2013).
  - PTSD is an anxiety disorder triggered by a traumatic event.
  - Symptoms include: nightmares, elevated heart rate and blood pressure (BP), and avoidance of reminders of the event.
  - Treatments include cognitive behavioral therapy, exposure therapy, eye movement desensitization and reprocessing (EMDR), and antidepressants.
  - Nursing considerations:
    - Notify provider if symptoms are noted.
    - Follow recommendations from therapists regarding communication and handling.
- Falls
  - Forty percent of stroke patients experience falls during the early rehabilitative phase; 22% sustain injuries as a result.
  - More common with hemi-neglect, cognitive impairment, sedatives, and more severe deficits

- Nursing considerations:
  - Call bells or some mechanism for the patient to summon help should be within reach on the unaffected side.
  - Ensure glasses, proper lighting, and nonskid footwear are in place when mobilizing.
  - Environmental adaptations to reduce risk for falling, such as handrails, grab bars, nonslip mats, raised toilet seats, limitation of throw rugs, elimination of clutter, and avoiding over fatigue
- Instruct patients and family members how to get up after a fall since injury during the attempt to get up is common, as well as danger of being stuck out of reach of phone or bell for extended periods of time.
- Malnutrition
  - At 2 to 3 weeks afterstroke, malnutrition is reported in 50% of severe stroke patients.
  - Nursing considerations:
    - Weight loss greater than 3 kg indicates need for close review of nutritional status.
    - If imbalance is suspected, monitor urinary output for color as well as amount in contrast to oral fluid intake.
    - Collaboration with SLP and dietician is essential to determine cause of malnutrition.
  - Treatment involves supplemental feedings and fluid intake.
- Spasticity
  - Occurs in up to 65% of stroke patients
  - Treatment involves stretching, splinting, and medications
    - Botulinum toxin injection into the spastic muscle has proven effective in improving range of motion (ROM) and preventing contractures when used for focal spasticity.
    - Oral baclofen, benzodiazepines, and tizanidine have been used for generalized spasticity, but their usefulness is limited secondary to sedative effects.

- – Intrathecal Baclofen can be administered with an implanted pump.
- ▪ Nursing considerations:
  - – Provide/encourage ROM exercises throughout the day; follow the therapist's recommendations, but it is not just the therapists' responsibility to do the exercises.
  - – Understand proper placement of splints and ensure they are used according to therapist's recommendations

FAMILY AND CAREGIVER SUPPORT

- • Family/caregiver stress and inability to continue to provide care are the leading causes of institutionalization of stroke patients.
- • There is an increased risk of depression, social isolation, health deterioration, and mortality
  - ▪ Depression prevalence up to 52%
  - ▪ Mortality increase of 63%
- • Nursing considerations:
  - ▪ Assessment of family/caregivers needs and concerns should be done on an ongoing basis.
  - ▪ Assessment tools are available for use throughout the rehabilitation process (Miller et al., 2010).

REHABILITATION TREATMENTS

- • Devices
  - ▪ Functional electrical stimulation therapy
    - – Electrodes placed on affected limb can cause movement of the limb; repetition can result in some degree of functional improvement.
    - – Upper extremity: Bioness (Ness) H200, Neuromove T
    - – Lower extremity: Bioness (Ness) H300, WalkAide
    - – Swallowing: VitalStim, Experia

- Dynamic splinting
  - For wrist and hand to mechanically assist in straightening
  - Saeboflex
- Partial body weight-supported treadmills (BWSTT)
  - Uses a harness to reduce weight bearing while providing practice walking
  - AutoAmbulator, Lokomat, LiteGait, SMART Balance Master
- Robotic therapy
  - Sophisticated exercise machines that guide the patient through repetitive movements
  - Upper extremity: InMotion 2 and 3, ReoGo, Amadeo, Myomo e100
  - Lower extremity: ReoAmbulator, Anklebot, PK100
- Therapies
  - Constraint-induced movement therapy (CIMT)
    - The unaffected arm is placed in a restrictive mitt to encourage use of the weak upper limb; classic therapy involves 6 hours, 5 days per week for a 2-week period.
  - Botulinum toxin (see "Spasticity" bulleted section on page 147)
    - Botox, Dysport, Myobloc
  - Brain stimulation
    - Repetitive stimulation over the area of infarction to enhance the brain's ability to rewire itself
    - Transcranial magnetic stimulation (TMS) and transcranial direct current stimulation (TDCS)
  - Virtual reality
    - Computerized artificial environment used to practice movements, improving arm and leg mobility and strength
    - "Wii-hab," or "Wii-habilitation," Armeo
  - Mental practice
    - Involves imagining movement of the affected limb, usually the arm, with aid of audio recording to facilitate focus
    - Effective as adjunct therapy to CIMT

- Mirror therapy
  - Use of mirror to create appearance of affected arm moving normally in a symmetric, two-armed activity; the patient is actually seeing the unaffected arm in the mirror.
- Cognitive therapy
  - Two general treatment approaches:
    - Retraining impaired cognitive skills—task-specific
    - Training strategies to compensate for impaired skills
  - Performed by a variety of health care disciplines—communication among team members is imperative to avoid omissions or duplication of services

FAST FACTS in a NUTSHELL

Overall, among stroke survivors, women over age 65 have greater disability than men; in fact they are half as likely to be independent in activities of daily living, even after controlling for age, race, education, and marital status (Go et al., 2013).

- Emerging strategies and research in stroke rehabilitation
  - National Institutes of Neurological Diseases and Stroke (NINDS)–sponsored clinical trials
    - Locomotor Experience Applied Post-Stroke (LEAPS)
      - Comparison of BWSTT with simple walking practice at 2-months and 6-months afterstroke
    - Interdisciplinary Comprehensive Arm Rehabilitation Evaluation (I-CARE)
      - Arm therapy called Accelerated Skills Acquisition Program (ASAP) that combines practice of tasks of the participant's choice compared to two standard types of therapy (customary arm therapy totaling 30 hours, and customary arm therapy for a duration indicated on the therapy prescription)

- Neural stem cell transplantation
  - Research has been ongoing regarding whether administration of intravenous (IV) stem cells can impact brain recovery and functional outcomes after stroke.
- Brain imaging as complement to therapies
  - Research indicates that positron emission tomography (PET) scan imaging in conjunction with therapy activity can provide a map of areas that light up with each therapy.
    - Implication is that it would facilitate a customized therapy plan of care
    - Limited application due to expense and not widely available
- Implantable nerve stimulators
  - Similar to the transcranial stimulation devices, but implantation onto the cortical surface
    - Eliminates need to keep head shaved as with transcranial device.
    - More direct stimulation of affected area
    - More invasive than transcranial
- Phosphodiesterase inhibitor—to determine whether there is facilitation of neurogenesis and synaptogenesis and improvement of regional blood flow in ischemic stroke

FAST FACTS in a NUTSHELL

Research trials in stroke rehabilitation are on the rise. Unfortunately, most research continues to be related to physical functional recovery. Cognitive deficits impact 65% of stroke patients and present barriers to rehabilitation, but very few research studies have been done related to cognitive deficits (Duncan, 2007). Experts agree that the nature of cognitive deficits and current evaluation methods make it very hard to establish distinct categories of patients for the purposes of research.

17

Secondary Prevention

Secondary prevention refers to a variety of treatments, procedures, medications, and lifestyle changes to reduce the risk of another vascular event—a stroke, transient ischemic attack (TIA), or myocardial infarction (MI). Of the 795,000 strokes that occur each year, approximately 25% are recurrent events. No one will argue that the cost of health care is becoming prohibitive, and without sweeping changes the costs will continue to rise. Experts have predicted a 129% increase in the cost of stroke care by 2030 (Ovbiagele et al., 2013). Therefore, hospitalization for stroke or TIA is the health care professional's opportunity to provide secondary prevention. For some patients, the hospital stay is their first comprehensive health assessment in some time. The procedures for secondary prevention have been discussed in Chapters 10 and 11. This chapter provides an overview of the risk factors, medications, nonacute treatments, and lifestyle changes that have been proven to reduce the risk of secondary stroke.

In this chapter, you will learn:

1. The most common risk factors for stroke
2. Recommendations for control and/or elimination of the risk factors for stroke

FAST FACTS in a NUTSHELL

Telemedicine, described in Chapter 12, plays an important role not only in emergency stroke care, but also in secondary prevention of stroke. Small hospitals, through the use of telestroke technology, now have neurological expert guidance in determining the etiology of the stroke, which is essential for customizing the plan of care to prevent another stroke—secondary prevention.

HYPERTENSION

- The most important preventable and treatable cause of stroke and TIA
- In 2003, the National Institutes of Health (NIH) changed the way we think about blood pressure (BP) (National Institutes of Health, 2003).
  - From a baseline of 115/75, the risk of heart attack and stroke doubles for every 20-point rise in systolic BP, or every 10-point rise in diastolic BP.
- Prehypertension: BP between 120/80 and 140/90; these levels were once considered normal.
  - *Twice* the risk of heart disease or stroke
- Hypertension: BP above 140/90
  - Four times the risk of heart disease or stroke
- Medications:
  - Angiotensin receptor blockers (ARB), angiotensin-converting enzyme (ACE) inhibitors, calcium channel blockers, beta blockers
  - Selection based on patient's comorbid conditions, age, and race
    - Caucasians respond better to ARBs

  – African Americans respond better to ACE Inhibitors plus diuretic
  – Diabetic patients—ACE inhibitors are preferred

DIABETES

- Diabetes affects 8% of the adult population in the United States (Furie et al., 2011).
  - Reported prevalence in the ischemic stroke population is up to 33%
  - Associated with patients with multiple lacunar strokes
- On entering red blood cells, glucose links up (or glycates) with hemoglobin; the more glucose present in the blood, the more hemoglobin gets glycated (Hgb A1C)
- Hgb A1C represents the average blood glucose control for the previous 2 to 3 months
  - Goal for Hgb A1C is less than 7%
- Medications: Insulin or oral agents

LIPIDS

- Low-density lipoprotein cholesterol (LDL-C) goal is less than 100 mg/dL; for patients with multiple risk factors, goal is less than 70 mg/dL
  - Medications:
    – Statins—most recommended in clinical guidelines for cholesterol reduction
    – Cholesterol absorption inhibitors
    – Bile acid suppressants
- High-density lipoprotein cholesterol (HDL-C) goal is greater than 60
- Triglycerides: goal is less than 150
  - Medications:
    – Fibrates and nicotinic acid—for combination of low HDL and high triglycerides

METABOLIC SYNDROME

- Presence of several physiological abnormalities, the combined effect of which increases the risk of vascular disease
  - Hypertriglyceridemia
  - Low HDL-C
  - Hypertension
  - Hyperglycemia
  - Increased waist circumference 102 cm or above in men, 88 cm or above in women)
- Present in 22% of adults and 40% to 50% of ischemic stroke patients
- Consequences are reduced peripheral glucose uptake (into muscle and fat), increased hepatic glucose production, and increased pancreatic insulin secretion (compensatory)

CAROTID ARTERY DISEASE

- Medical management and prevention include blood pressure control, antithrombotics, and statins
- Intervention is indicated for stroke patients with stenosis of greater than 50%.
  - Timing is recommended to be within 2 weeks of diagnosis
  - See Chapter 8 for a discussion of carotid endarterectomy and carotid artery stenting.

VERTEBROBASILAR DISEASE

- Medical management and prevention include BP control, antithrombotics, and statins
- Interventions includes endarterectomy, bypass grafting, arterial transposition, and stenting
  - Selection of intervention is patient/provider specific and primarily based on degree of stenosis and symptoms

ATRIAL FIBRILLATION

- Occurs in 10% of people over 80 years of age
- Associated with more severe strokes and poorer clinical outcomes
- Stratification of risk allows for individualized medical therapy
  - CHADS$_2$ score:

    - Cardiac failure   1 point
    - Hypertension   1 point
    - Age   1 point
    - Diabetes   1 point
    - Prior stroke or TIA   2 points

  - Patients with score of 0 receive antithrombotics; score of 1 or above receive anticoagulation (Gage et al., 2001)
- Other treatments are discussed in Chapter 10.

CARDIOMYOPATHY

- Affects approximately 10% of ischemic stroke patients
- Causes ventricular dilatation and decreased cardiac output (left ventricular ejection fraction [LVEF])—predisposes patients to hypertension and atrial fibrillation
- Treatment includes anticoagulation for ejection fraction greater than 30% or evidence of ventricular thrombus.

VALVULAR HEART DISEASE

- Provides a nidus for clot formation, thus creating risk for cardioembolic stroke
- Treatment includes antithrombotic therapy for non-rheumatic valve disease; anticoagulant therapy for those with rheumatic mitral valve disease

- Infectious endocarditis treatment involves anticoagulation and antibiotic therapy
- Prosthetic valves require anticoagulation; addition of aspirin if stroke or TIA occurred with therapeutic international normalized ratio (INR)

ARTERIAL DISSECTION

- Mechanism of arterial dissection was discussed in Chapter 5
- Treatment involves antithrombotic therapy for a minimum of 3 to 6 months
  - If an event stroke or TIA occurred while on antithrombotic therapy, may add anticoagulation therapy
- If recurrent stroke or TIA was due to dissection, endovascular stenting may be considered

DIET AND LIFESTYLE

- Healthy diet:
  - DASH diet (dietary approaches to stop hypertension)—reduction in dietary sodium to 2,300 mg a day or less; also includes low consumption of animal fat and processed foods; limited caffeine
  - Limit: red meat, refined carbohydrates, and sugary drinks
  - Focus on: plant foods and whole grains, fruits and vegetables, low-fat dairy
- Regular physical activity: minimum of 30 minutes 1 to 3 days/week
- Healthy weight: body mass index (BMI) less than 25
- Stop smoking
- Limit alcohol: two drinks or less per day for men; one drink per day for women
- Manage stress
- Take medications as prescribed

===== *FAST FACTS in a NUTSHELL*

There are no standards or guidelines for when, or how often, a stroke patient should be seen after discharge from the acute care hospital, and whether the patient should be seen by a specialist. There have been some research studies done to determine the optimal pattern for follow-up, but no one protocol has been found to be superior to others. All seem to agree, however, that follow-up after acute stroke is essential not only in preventing recurrent stroke, but also in preventing readmission.

Follow-Up Visits/Phone Calls

- Primary care physician (PCP): within 1 to 2 weeks after discharge
- Neurologist or neurosurgeon: within 2 to 4 weeks after discharge
  - Some specialists see the patients again at 3 months, 6 months, and 1 year depending on the status of the patient and need for closer monitoring.
- Phone calls are made for a variety of purposes:
  - To provide support and answer questions: usually done within 1 week
  - To gather outcome information: usually done after 1 month and at varying intervals
  - To gather patient satisfaction information: usually done after 1 month to avoid interfering with hospital survey of patient satisfaction

Avoiding Silos

- Individual providers conducting independent follow-ups with patients are a recipe for disaster
- Communication is needed between PCP and specialist

- The AVAIL (Adherence eValuation After Ischemic stroke – Longitudinal) Registry reported in 2011 that of the 2,880 patients enrolled, the most common reason for nonadherence to the discharge medical regimen was discontinuation of medications by the PCP (Bushnell et al., 2011).
- The PROTECT (Preventing Recurrence of Thromboembolic Events Through Coordinated Treatment) study reported that 6 months after discharge, two thirds of stroke patients had discontinued their antithrombotic medication; a majority of these patients reported that their PCP had told them they didn't need it.
- Pilot programs have shown promising improvements with the following:
  – Handoff letter that the patient carries to the PCP
    • Contains information about the need for continuation of specific medications that the PCP may not have been aware of

FAST FACTS in a NUTSHELL

Most poststroke follow-up tools focus on compliance with medications, follow-up appointments, exercise, and diet. Although these are important, they do not capture the "intangibles" such as depression, anxiety, or changes in cognition that impact not only the patient's ability to be compliant, but the patient's quality of life as well. Attention to such long-term problems that occur poststroke have been difficult to measure. With the challenges of high readmission and mortality rates after stroke, a tool that would prompt providers to address these issues as well as provide a tool to track actions taken, could be quite effective in improving follow-up care, and patients' ability to comply with their plans of care.

- – Concrete, formalized follow-up plan
- – Patient tracking logs and calendars
- Get With the Guidelines (GWTG) 30-Day Follow-Up Form
  - – Established by the American Heart Association/ American Stroke Association in 2003
  - – Facilitates a standardized approach for health care providers to address compliance with the plan of care poststroke
  - – Standardized tool for tracking compliance and outcomes

THE POSTSTROKE CHECKLIST

- Established by the Global Stroke Community Advisory Panel (GSCAP) in 2011
  - Medical experts from seven countries
  - Endorsed by the World Stroke Organization (WSO)

Identification of 11 key poststroke problems that are not routinely addressed in poststroke follow-up visits, but were amenable to effective interventions (Philp et al., 2013).

- Simple, easy-to-use, free tool (Figure 17.1)
  - Facilitates a standardized approach for health care providers to identify problems
    - – A concise checklist that prompts the provider to address each topic
  - Facilitates appropriate referrals for treatment
  - Provides a standardized tool for tracking the provider's response to identified problems
    - – Correlation between patient outcomes and poststroke management may demonstrate effectiveness of specific interventions
  - Excellent adjunct to tools such as the GWTG 30-Day Follow-Up Form
  - Available for download at http://www.world-stroke .org/advocacy/post-stroke-checklist

POST-STROKE CHECKLIST (PSC):
IMPROVING LIFE AFTER STROKE

This Post-Stroke Checklist (PSC) has been developed to help healthcare professionals identify post-stroke problems amenable to treatment and subsequent referral. The PSC is a brief and easy-to-use tool, intended for completion with the patient and the help of a caregiver, if necessary. **PSC administration provides a standardized approach for the identification of long-term problems in stroke survivors and facilitates appropriate referral** for treatment.

INSTRUCTIONS FOR USE:

Please ask the patient each numbered question and indicate the answer in the "response" section. In general, if the response is NO, update the patient record and review at next assessment. If the response is YES, follow-up with the appropriate action.

1. SECONDARY PREVENTION

| Since your stroke or last assessment, have you received any advice on health related life style changes or medications for preventing another stroke? | **NO** | If **NO**, refer to a Primary Care Physician or Stroke Neurologist for risk factor assessment and treatment if appropriate |
| | **YES** | Observe Progress |

2. ACTIVITIES OF DAILY LIVING (ADL)

| | **NO** | Observe Progress |
| Since your stroke or last assessment, **are you finding it more difficult to take** care of yourself? | **YES** | Do you have difficulty dressing, washing and/or bathing? Do you have difficulty preparing hot drinks and/or meals? Do you have difficulty getting outside? | If **YES** to any, refer to Primary Care Physician, Rehabilitation Physician or an appropriate therapist (i.e. OT or PT) for further assessment |

3. MOBILITY

	NO	Observe Progress
Since your stroke or last assessment, **are you finding it more difficult to walk** or move safely from bed to chair?	**YES**	Are you continuing to receive rehabilitation therapy?	If **YES**, update patient record and review at next assessment
			If **NO**, refer to Primary Care Physician, Rehabilitation Physician or an appropriate therapist (i.e. OT or PT) for further assessment

4. SPASTICITY

	NO	Observe Progress
Since your stroke or last assessment, do you have increasing stiffness in your arms, hands, and/or legs?	**YES**	Is this interfering with activities of daily living, sleep or causing pain?	If **YES**, refer to a physician with an interest in post-stroke spasticity (i.e. Rehabilitation Physician or Stroke Neurologist) for further assessment
			If **NO**, update patient record and review at next assessment

FIGURE 17.1 Post-Stroke Checklist.

5. PAIN

Since your stroke or last assessment, do you have any *new* pain?

NO → Observe Progress

YES → If **YES**, refer to a physician with an interest in post-stroke pain for further assessment and diagnosis

6. INCONTINENCE

Since your stroke or last assessment, are you having *more* of a problem controlling your bladder or bowels?

NO → Observe Progress

YES → If **YES**, refer to Healthcare Provider with an interest in incontinence

7. COMMUNICATION

Since your stroke or last assessment, **are you finding it *more* difficult to communicate with others?**

NO → Observe Progress

YES → If **YES**, refer to specialist Speech and Language Pathologist for further assessment

8. MOOD

Since your stroke or last assessment, do you feel *more* anxious or depressed?

NO → Observe Progress

YES → If **YES**, refer to a Physician or Psychologist with an interest in post-stroke mood changes for further assessment

9. COGNITION

Since your stroke or last assessment, **are you finding it *more* difficult to think, concentrate, or remember things?**

NO → Observe Progress

YES → Does this interfere with activity or participation? → If **YES**, refer to a Physician or Psychologist with an interest in post-stroke cognition for further assessment

If **NO**, update patient record and review at next assessment

10. LIFE AFTER STROKE

Since your stroke or last assessment, **are you finding things important to you *more* difficult to carry out** (e.g. leisure activities, hobbies, work)

NO → Observe Progress

YES → If **YES**, refer to a local stroke support group or a stroke association (i.e. The American Stroke Association or National Stroke Association)

11. RELATIONSHIP WITH FAMILY

Since your stroke or last assessment, has your relationship with your family become *more* **difficult or stressed?**

NO → Observe Progress

YES → If **YES**, schedule next Primary Care visit with patient and family member. If family member is present refer to a local stroke support group

Adapted from: Philip I, et al. Development of a Poststroke Checklist to Standardize Follow-up Care for Stroke Survivors. *Journal of Stroke and Cerebrovascular Diseases.* December 2012.
Endorsed by the World Stroke Organization to support improved stroke survivor follow-up and care

APC10i513

FIGURE 17.1 Post-Stroke Checklist. (*continued*)

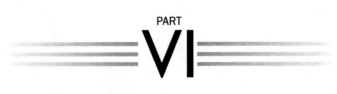

PART

VI

Primary Prevention Essentials

18

Primary Prevention

Of the 795,000 people annually in the United States who have stroke, approximately 610,000 are first events. If people continue with the lifestyles that increase the risk of vascular disease and stroke, the incidence of stroke will continue to rise. Surveys of people at risk have indicated that major stroke is viewed as worse than death. Yet in 2012, the Get With the Guidelines (GWTG) Stroke registry, with over 2.5 million patients registered, showed that only 25% of stroke patients arrived at the hospital within the 3-hour treatment window for intravenous (IV) tissue plasminogen activator (tPA), with over 60% arriving more than 9 hours from the time they were last known well. Even with the exciting developments in acute stroke treatment, if people ignore the symptoms of stroke, we will continue to have challenges in providing the acute treatments to more people. Therefore, the most effective strategy for improving the burden of stroke is to prevent stroke from happening in the first place.

In this chapter, you will learn:

1. Assessment of risk factors for first stroke
2. Target populations
3. Community education strategies

FAST FACTS in a NUTSHELL

Except for the headache associated with hemorrhagic stroke, symptoms of stroke do not hurt. Pain is a great motivator for seeking treatment, and its absence makes it possible for stroke patients to adopt a "wait and see" and "hope this goes away" mentality. Precious time is lost, limiting the acute treatment options available.

RISK-FACTOR ASSESSMENT

- Classified as nonmodifiable, modifiable, or potentially modifiable (Goldstein et al., 2011)
- Nonmodifiable risk factors are few: age, gender, low birth weight, race/ethnicity, and genetics
  - Individuals with one or more of these risk factors are advised to pay close attention to the modifiable risk factors
    - Age: Risk doubles with each decade after age 55
    - Gender: Men have a higher incidence of stroke than women, except for ages 35 to 44, and over 85 years of age
    - Low birth weight: Risk is more than double for babies with birth weight less than 2,500 g (5 lbs 8 oz)
    - Race/ethnicity: Blacks and Hispanic/Latino Americans have higher incidence and mortality rates than Whites
    - Genetics: Coagulopathies and intracranial aneurysms have been shown to have familial tendencies;

Marfan syndrome, sickle cell disease and Fabry disease are associated with increased stroke risk
- Modifiable risk factors include:
  - Hypertension
  - Cigarette smoking
  - Diabetes
  - Dyslipidemia
  - Atrial fibrillation
  - Valvular heart disease
  - Carotid stenosis
  - Postmenopausal hormone therapy
  - Oral contraceptives
  - Diet/nutrition
  - Physical inactivity
  - Obesity/body fat distribution
- Potentially modifiable risk factors include:
  - Migraine, particularly migraine with aura: possible link between migraines and patent foramen ovales (PFOs) due to paradoxical embolism via the PFO; possible increase in platelet activation and platelet–leukocyte aggregation increasing risk for emboli formation
  - Metabolic syndrome: the presence of three or more of the following: abdominal obesity, high triglycerides, low high-density lipoprotein (HDL), hypertension, and hyperglycemia
    – Associated with insulin resistance, inflammation, diabetes, and heart disease
  - Alcohol consumption: heavy alcohol use (more than 21 drinks per week) is associated with hypertension, hypercoagulability, reduced cerebral blood flow, and atrial fibrillation
    – Recommendation is two drinks or less per day for men and one drink or less per day for women
  - Drug abuse: cocaine, amphetamines, and heroin are linked to hypertension, cerebral vasospasm, vasculitis, infectious endocarditis, increased blood viscosity, and intracerebral hemorrhage (ICH)

- Sleep-disordered breathing: loud snoring and sleep apnea are associated with increased carotid atherosclerosis, cardiomyopathy, atrial fibrillation, and hypertension
- Hypercoagulability: associated with arterial thrombosis
- Inflammation: chronic conditions such as rheumatoid arthritis and lupus have been associated with initiation, growth, and destabilization of atherosclerotic plaque.
- Infection: chronic infection with bacteria such as *Helicobacter pylori* can promote atherosclerosis.
- Hyperhomocysteinemia: increased levels of the amino acidhomocysteine have been associated with atherosclerosis.
- Elevated lipoprotein (a): similar to low-density lipoprotein (LDL), associated with atherosclerosis and thrombosis

- Numerous first-time stroke risk assessment tools have been used, but experts agree that an ideal, comprehensive tool does not yet exist.
  - Framingham Stroke Risk Profile is one of most widely used
    - Analyzes risk factors and provides a gender-specific, 10-year cumulative stroke risk

FAST FACTS in a NUTSHELL

Adherence rates for treatment and control of risk factors such as hypertension for primary prevention are improving. Currently, 61% of people with hypertension are being treated, unfortunately only 35% of those treated actually have their hypertension controlled (Goldstein et al., 2011). As long as the hypertension continues to be over 120/80, vascular damage is occurring and the risk of stroke continues.

OPPORTUNITIES FOR PREVENTIVE HEALTH SERVICES

- Emergency departments (ED)
  - Visits to the ED are increasing due to several factors: (a) increased number of people without insurance, (b) lack of primary care providers (PCPs), (c) decreased availability of medical specialists, and (c) inadequate preventive and chronic care management
  - Point of contact and opportunity to screen and initiate treatment for patients with hypertension, diabetes, atrial fibrillation, and other risk factors such as smoking and alcohol and drug abuse
- Primary care practices
  - Strategies aimed at provider practice to improve adherence with guideline recommendations include: physician education, audit and feedback of practice patterns, physician and patient profiling
  - Strategies aimed at systems are thought to be more effective; these include: computer-based clinical reminders, electronic medical records, support personnel to implement preventive health protocols, and separate clinics devoted to screening and preventive services.

TARGET POPULATIONS

- Unique differences by race
  - Blacks have the highest incidence of stroke in the United States (191/100,000)
    - Uncontrolled hypertension is the most common cause
    - Strokes tend to be more severe, with higher degree of deficits
    - Continues to be the second leading cause of death for Blacks
  - Hispanics have the second highest incidence (149/100,000)

- Uncontrolled diabetes and hypertension are the top causes
- Between 2010 and 2050, the incidence is expected to rise from 16% to 30.2%
  - Access to care has been identified as a barrier for both Blacks and Hispanics
    - Socioeconomic status, fewer community resources, and lack of knowledge about stroke symptoms and risk factors have been identified
  - Whites have the third highest incidence (88/100,000) (Heart Disease and Stroke Statistics, 2013)
- Unique differences by gender

Women

- Natural menopause prior to age 42 may indicate increased risk for ischemic stroke
- Birth control pill use
  - Older, higher dose estrogen pills carry three times the risk of ischemic stroke
  - Newer, lower dose estrogen pills still carry twice the risk
    - Risk of stroke is outweighed by the benefit of preventing pregnancy, which itself carries risk of stroke
  - Combination of smoking and birth control pill use greatly increases risk for stroke
- Postpartum period of 6 weeks associated with increased risk of stroke, particularly for Blacks and older women of all races
- In 2012, the American Stroke Association (ASA) reported that 100,000 women under age 65 suffered a stroke
- Stroke is the second leading cause of death for women

Men

- Hypertension
- Abdominal obesity
- Maternal history of death from stroke
- The Stroke Belt
  - Southeast United States: highest mortality rate from stroke

- 20% higher than rest of the United States
- "Buckle" refers to coastal North Carolina, South Carolina, and Georgia
  • Highest mortality rate of the Stroke Belt: 40% higher than national average
■ Cause is combination of race, low socioeconomic status, and limited access to care
• Children and stroke
  ■ Incidence is reported as 4.6 to 6.4/100,000 (Heart Disease & Stroke Statistics, 2013)
    - Boys have slighter higher incidence than girls
    - Blacks have a twofold higher incidence than Whites
  ■ Half of all childhood strokes are hemorrhagic, with most common cause being aneurysm or arteriovenous malformation (AVM) rupture.
  ■ Most common cause of arterial ischemic stroke is cerebral arteriopathy and sickle cell disease.
  ■ Risk factors such as hyperlipidemia, obesity, and type 2 diabetes have been increasing in adolescents since 1995.

═══════════════════════════*FAST FACTS in a NUTSHELL*

Children are ideal for targeting stroke awareness and prevention education for several reasons: (a) risk factors for stroke begin in childhood, (b) increasing numbers of children are being raised by their grandparents—up 16% since 2005 (Scommegna, 2012), and (c) children have no preconceived notion, or dread, of the word "stroke," which is something that seems to develop through adulthood. Simple, age-appropriate education can be effective for this population.

COMMUNITY EDUCATION

• Know your community and tailor education materials to the message you want to give.

- Resources and materials
  - ASA and American Heart Association (AHA): www
    .strokeassociation.org and www.americanheart.org
    - Community awareness resources
  - National Stroke Association (NSA): www.stroke.org
    - Stroke awareness resources: www.strokeawareness
      .com
      - Collaboration with American College of Emer-
        gency Physicians
  - The Internet Stroke Center: www.strokecenter.org/
    patients/caregivers.htm
    - Stroke awareness resources
  - Each of these sites offers a variety of materials, some
    are customizable, many are free.

VENUES

- Health fairs
  - Message should be simple and concise; avoid pam-
    phlets and brochures
    - Single-page tools for risk assessment are ideal
      - ASA's Family Tree Risk Assessment (part of
        Power to End Stroke campaign)
      - NSA's Stroke Risk Scorecard
    - Time for discussion is very limited
  - Get them to stop at your table; be interactive
    - Game wheel for asking stroke questions
    - Colorful display with interactive messaging (lift
      tabs for answers)
    - Offer "prize" for correct answer; instead of sim-
      ply handing out magnets, pens, and so forth, give
      them as a prize for answering questions from the
      game wheel or display board
  - Always include some information about children and
    stroke (available at resources listed above); adults are
    always interested in children's health
  - Community groups
    - Churches, clubs, teams, employers

- Lecture format or screenings
- Tailor to your audience, but always include something about children and stroke
- Children
  - Turn them into "Stroke Detectives!"
    - Teach them the F.A.S.T. (face, arm, speech, time) acronym and the importance of calling 911
      - Stroke Heroes Act Fast is an excellent tool; available at www.mass.gov/eohhs/gov/departments/dph/programs/community-health/heart-disease-stroke/stroke-heroes-act-fast.html
    - Review healthy lifestyle choices: healthy food choices and physical activity
    - Stroke deficit reenactments: Let the children experience tying their shoe, loading a backpack, and so forth, with one arm in a sling; obstacle course with leg weights on one leg; reading flash cards with hemianopia glasses
  - Schools, after school programs, summer camps, churches, Scout troops, teams
  - Interactive, 30 minutes or less is ideal
  - Game wheel, making FAST bookmarks/doorhangers, and so on; coloring activities, crossword puzzles, word searches
  - Send them home with a simple letter to their parents with the message that their children became Stroke Detectives having learned about FAST and healthy lifestyle choices; parents will pay more attention to messages about their children's health.

MEASURING IMPACT

- Very difficult to measure primary prevention effectiveness: How do you know whether someone avoided a stroke because he or she changed a risk factor?
- Track community incidence of stroke: long-term strategy

- Hospital tracking: effective community outreach should result in an increase in:
  - Percentage of patients who arrive by emergency medical serices (EMS)
  - Percentage who arrive within the treatment window
  - Percentage who received IV tPA and/or advanced intervention
- Survey of community groups regarding stroke awareness before and after educational session

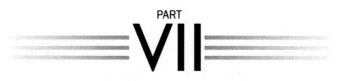

PART

VII

Evidence-Based Practice

19

Connecting Data to Clinical Practice

Historically, nurses performed patient care functions they learned in school or were shown on the job by a colleague who had been doing it a long time. They followed provider orders that were based on whatever the provider had learned in school, or through experience. Standardized orders were created for the providers, based on their preferences, for the purpose of saving them writing out each order and to eliminate the issue of illegible handwriting. Stroke research data and clinical practice guidelines became available in the 1990s, but existed in a different realm from that of the frontline bedside nurses. Many providers grumbled that the idea of standardizing orders based on research evidence represented "cookbook" medicine and could not possibly be good for each individual patient. But time and outcomes evidence have proven them wrong; organizations that have incorporated the evidence-based guidelines into their orders and protocols have shown improved patient outcomes (Schwamm et al., 2010). Since 2008, the Centers for Medicare & Medicaid Services (CMS) has linked hospital reimbursement to quality-of-care standards. Bundled payment initiatives are making hospitals accountable for the entire continuum of care, beyond hospital discharge.

In this chapter you will learn:

1. Performance improvement does not have to be a dirty word
2. Strategies for bedside nurses to drive care changes
3. Data use
4. Strategies to build a case for the stroke coordinator role

PERFORMANCE IMPROVEMENT, ALSO KNOWN AS QUALITY IMPROVEMENT

Since the Institute of Medicine (IOM) published *To Err is Human: Building a Safer Health System* in 1999, and hospitals instituted quality-improvement initiatives based on the evidence provided, health care has not been the same. The good news is that health care has not been the same; change was needed.

- Performance improvement (PI) is the process of evaluating outcomes related to the current process and making changes to improve the likelihood of better outcomes
  - Plan, Do, Check, Act (PDCA)
    - Plan an intervention or change in practice/process
    - Implement the planned change
    - Evaluate the results of the changed practice/process
    - Act on that result: Either maintain the change or make further adjustments
    - Continuous-cycle process until the outcome meets/exceeds the goal
  - Whether we realize it or not, PI is done virtually every day in every organization
    - Sometimes referred to as "workarounds," but if a process is altered and the outcomes are monitored, that is PI

BEDSIDE NURSES CAN DRIVE CARE CHANGES

- Nurses are in the best position to know what their patients need to achieve best outcomes.
  - Observations made during daily care

- Review of literature and attendance at nursing conferences, seminars, professional association meetings
- Nursing department practice councils, multidisciplinary team meetings
- A plan is needed: population and process to be measured, time frame, data-collection tool
- Evidence can be gathered to support a hypothesis or to support a proposed change
  - Data can be gathered over a short period of time, for a specific target population
  - Does not have to be a large, formal research protocol
    - Tracking time from failed swallow screen to start of enteral nutrition
      - Nurses at a community hospital had observed that their neurologic patients who could not take oral nutrition waited longer than 3 days for enteral orders to be placed.
        - They gathered evidence over a period of 3 months that the intensivists were not ordering nutritional support for more than 4 days, a fact that the intensivists had consistently denied prior to seeing the evidence.
    - Hypothermia
      - Tracking time from initiation of hypothermia to attainment of goal temperature
      - Time to control of shiver: patient report, observation
      - Time from initiation of rewarm to attainment of normal temperature
- Small tests of change have been proven to be effective in demonstrating process change efficacy
  - Blood pressure (BP) management post intravenous (IV) tissue plasminogen activator (tPA)
    - Nurses at an academic medical center had observed that the average time from identification of a BP outside parameters until control was greater than 60 minutes; research suggests that for each 10 minutes of hypertension above the

180 mmHg recommended, the likelihood of hemorrhagic transformation increased by 59%.

- They worked through their multidisciplinary team to develop an algorithm that would provide for treatment of hypertension with as-needed medication/dose prior to notification of the provider; the agreed-on time frame was to be 3 months, and only in the post-IV tPA population.
- Results were that the average time from identification of hypertension to attainment of goal dropped to under 30 minutes.
- The algorithm has been expanded for use for all ischemic stroke patients.

FAST FACTS in a NUTSHELL

Benchmarking has been defined as the search for industry best practice that leads to superior performance (Camp, 1989). Organizations determine what best practices have been reported, then establish performance improvement goals based on that practice. Internal benchmarking involves comparison within an organization, either among departments or over time. For example, aspiration pneumonia rates among different intensive care units (ICUs) for a specified time frame, or aspiration pneumonia rates for a single ICU from one year to another. External benchmarking involves comparison with other competing organizations or national/international standards. The purpose of benchmarking is to determine whether an organization has the opportunity for improvement or a cause to celebrate best practice.

DATABASE USE

- Requires entry of patient-specific data points; usually done by, or overseen by, a stroke program coordinator

- Internal database
  - List of stroke patients along with key data points such as admission/discharge dates, discharge disposition, costs/case, complication rates, and so forth
  - Various tools utilized, from paper to Excel, Access, and so forth
  - Provides mechanism for tracking and trending of that organization's population
- External database
  - Tool with templates for entering patient-specific data points
  - Examples are Get With the Guidelines (GWTG), Midas and Coverdell, among others
    - A recent publication summarizes value of disease-based registries in improving quality of care (Ellrodt et al., 2013).
  - Provides mechanism for tracking and trending of organization's population
  - Benefit is that a database also allows for comparison to other organizations; examples are provided below

BUILDING THE CASE FOR A STROKE PROGRAM COORDINATOR

FAST FACTS in a NUTSHELL

Since 2000, when the Brain Attack Coalition first published its Recommendations for the Establishment of Primary Stroke Centers, many hospitals took a new look at the way they provided stroke care. Some recognized the need for a nurse coordinator to oversee the various aspects of stroke care, but unfortunately many have been slow in this realization. In the current financial environment, with hospitals tightening their belts, a comprehensive approach with data as evidence will help to get the attention of the administration.

- Cost–benefit analysis
  - The cost of salary, equipment (computer), software, or database
  - Payer mix (percentage that is Medicare, managed care, etc.), reimbursement for stroke and transient ischemic attacks (TIA) MS-DRGs (Medicare severity–diagnosis-related groups) (61–72) and cost of care per inpatient day
- Benefits of dedicated program coordinator
  - Adherence to standards: core measures, quality measures
  - Education for staff, not just nurses but also computed tomography (CT) techs, lab personnel, emergency medical services (EMS)
  - Community outreach activities to raise stroke awareness
  - Interdisciplinary team facilitation/communication
  - Concurrent review of cases facilitating real-time feedback to staff
  - Maintenance of database with ability to benchmark organizational performance and outcomes to other organizations
- Data give power!
  - Graphs and tables provide visual evidence of compliance with best practice standards and guidelines for care
    - Average length of stay (LOS), mortality rates, discharge disposition, complication rates
    - Report cards to providers (blinded) showing adherence to guidelines can be very powerful (Figure 19.1)
    - Showing compliance to a measure over time, with key action steps indicated along the way, demonstrates the effect of the action (Figure 19.2).
    - Comparison of compliance to a measure linked to the complication rate or associated outcome can also be powerful (Figure 19.3).
    - Showing the Door-to-Needle (D2N) times for an organization (Figure 19.4).
    - With the D2N time goal of less than 60 minutes, it may be helpful to break that time frame down

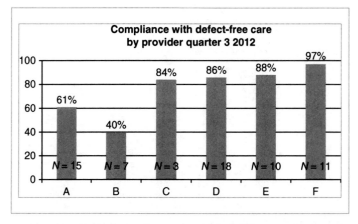

FIGURE 19.1 Report card for providers.

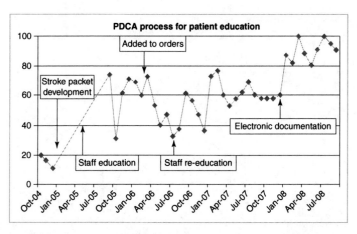

FIGURE 19.2 Compliance over time, with key actions to show impact.

into two key parts: (a) door-to-decision = the time from arrival to placement of order for thrombolytic, and (b) decision-to-needle = the time from order placement to time of thrombolytic administration. Goals can be set for each; for instance, making the door-to-decision goal of 30 minutes

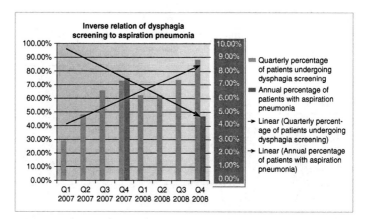

FIGURE 19.3 Compliance with dysphagia screening related to incidence of aspiration pneumonia.

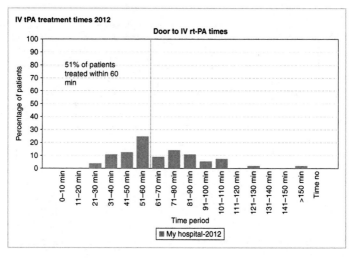

FIGURE 19.4 D2N times from one organization.

and the decision-to-needle goal of 15 minutes sets the pace for D2N to be less than 60 minutes (Figure 19.5).

– Comparison of D2N times with other hospitals and other Primary Stroke Centers (Figure 19.6)

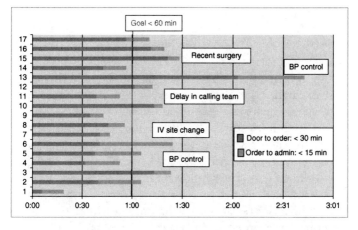

FIGURE 19.5 Door-to-Needle times graph.

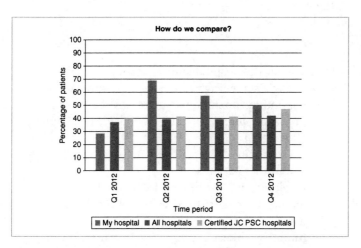

FIGURE 19.6 D2N times compared with other organizations.

FAST FACTS in a NUTSHELL

For years there has been inconsistency in how IV tPA treatment rates are reported. The early trials and publications generally utilized the total number of ischemic stroke patients as the denominator with the number of treated patients as the numerator. But critics have said that since most stroke patients do not arrive within the tPA treatment window, the denominator should only be the number of ischemic stroke patients who arrive within the 4.5-hour window. Many organizations have utilized that model for reporting. A recent publication by Kruyt et al. (2013) has provided evidence to support the proposal for establishment of a uniform reporting mechanism, using the 4.5-hour window as the denominator.

- Evidence for the hospital administration
  - Dysphagia screening reduces aspiration pneumonia
    - Aspiration pneumonia increases LOS, cost of care, and mortality rate, and decreases patient satisfaction
      - Decreasing LOS will facilitate bed availability for other patients
    - Difference in cost of care for aspiration pneumonia has been calculated to be 20% to 30% higher (two hospitals' data)
    - Initiatives like CMS Quality Initiative (present-on-admission criteria)
      - No reimbursement for care if pneumonia occurred during the hospital stay; can be difficult to prove that aspiration occurred with the stroke event prior to arrival; usually diagnosed more than 48 hours after admission.
    - Effective bedside screening by nurses has been shown to reduce aspiration pneumonia by over 50% (Hinchey, 2005).

- Development of a screening tool, protocol, education of staff, implementation of process, and monitoring of compliance and outcomes are part of the stroke nurse coordinator's role.
- Patients treated with IV tPA have 30% improved outcomes at 3 months.
  - The use of IV tPA has been shown to reduce overall costs of care (Demaerschalk et al., 2012).
  - Adherence to stroke center standards has demonstrated a significant increase in the number of patients who receive tPA.
  - In 2005, diagnosis-related group (DRG) 559 established increasing reimbursements to hospitals by approximately $6,000 per stroke patient if tPA is administered.
  - Documentation by provider of consideration/reason for not administering tPA is required, and often not done.
  - Development of the protocol, education of staff, implementation of process, and monitoring of compliance and outcomes are part of the stroke nurse coordinator's role.

Appendix
50 Neuroscience Terms

1. **Agnosia**—Failure to recognize stimuli when the appropriate sensory systems are functioning adequately; commonly occurs in visual, tactile, and auditory forms

2. **Antithrombotics**—Medications that prevent clot formation; two classes are anticoagulants and antiplatelet agents

3. **Aphasia**—Loss of ability to use language and to communicate thoughts verbally or in writing; receptive: inability to understand; expressive: inability to speak/write

4. **Ataxia**—Uncoordination or clumsiness of movement that is not the result of muscular weakness; it is caused by vestibular, cerebellar, or sensory disorders

5. **Aura**—Subjective sensation preceding a paroxysmal attack; may precede migraines or seizures and can be psychic or sensory in nature

6. **Clonic**—Alternating contraction and relaxation of muscles

7. **Collateral circulation**—Circulation of blood established through enlargement of minor vessels and anastomosis of vessels with those of adjacent parts when a major vein or artery is functionally impaired (as by obstruction)

8. **Comorbid conditions**—Presence of one or more disorders in addition to the primary disorder; for example, a stroke patients with diabetes and hypertension—these are comorbid conditions

9. **Contralateral**—Originating in, or affecting, the opposite side of the body

10. **Decerebrate**—Posture characterized by a rigid— possibly arched—spine, rigidly extended arms and legs, and plantar flexion; indicative of a brainstem lesion

11. **Decorticate**—Posture characterized by a rigid spine, inwardly flexed arms, extended and internally rotated legs, and plantar flexion; indicative of a brainstem lesion

12. **Delirium**—Mental confusion and excitement characterized by disorientation for time and place, usually with illusions and hallucinations; possible causes are fever, shock, exhaustion, anxiety, or drug overdose

13. **Dementia**—An acquired, generalized, and often progressive impairment of cognitive function that affects the content, but not the level, of consciousness; may indicate pathology affecting the cerebral cortex, its subcortical connections, or both

14. **Diplopia**—Double vision; may indicate pathology involving the cranial nerves, eyeballs, cerebellum, cerebrum, or meninges

15. **Dissection**—Separation of the layers of an arterial or venous wall resulting in reduced lumen and possibly complete occlusion

16. **Dysphagia**—Difficulty swallowing or inability to swallow

17. **Dysphasia**—Impaired ability to communicate with verbal or written language; seldom used in clinical care, as

aphasia has come to be used to represent not only the inability to communicate, but also the impaired ability to communicate; dysphasia is often confused with dysphagia

18. **Fissure**—Deep cleft or groove between segments of the cerebral cortex; larger than sulcus

19. **Grey matter**—Largest portion of the brain; neuronal cell bodies and glial cells in the cortex and deep nuclei process information originating in the sensory organs or in other grey matter regions

20. **Gyrus** (plural is **gyri**)—Prominent convolutions on the surface of the cerebral hemispheres

21. **Hemianopia**—Loss of half of the visual field; homonymous hemianopia means that both right visual fields or both left visual fields are lost

22. **Hemiparesis**—Weakness affecting only one side of the body; may indicate an intracranial structural lesion

23. **Hemiplegia**—Paralysis affecting only one side of the body; may indicate pathology of upper motor neurons

24. **Hemorrhagic transformation**—Also called hemorrhagic conversion; that is, leakage of blood from vessels in the ischemic stroke bed; the presence of blood "transforms" an ischemic stroke into a hemorrhagic stroke on imaging, but improved imaging makes it possible to differentiate a primary hemorrhage from an ischemic stroke with hemorrhagic transformation

25. **Hyperreflexia**—Abnormally intense response to a stimulus; may indicate a lesion of the upper motor neurons and suggests lack of cortical control over the reflex

26. **Ictal**—Pertaining to or caused by a sudden attack such as acute epilepsy

27. **Infarction**—Irreversible damage or death of tissue

28. **Intima**—Innermost lining of an artery or vein

29. **Intrathecal**—Introduction of substance into the subarachnoid space of the brain or spinal cord; certain drugs are given this way to avoid the blood–brain barrier

30. **Ipsilateral**—Originating in or affecting the same side of the body

31. **Ischemia**—Insufficient blood flow to meet metabolic demand; if not corrected, leads to hypoxia and infarction

32. **Myelin**—White fatty material that encloses the axons of myelinated nerve fibers; acts as an insulator, increasing the speed of transmission of nerve signals

33. **Myoclonic**—Twitching or clonic spasm of a muscle or group of muscles

34. **Nerve palsy**—Neurologic defect caused by dysfunction of nerve that controls that part of body; for example, third cranial nerve palsy is manifested by limited eye movements and ptosis

35. **Nystagmus**—Involuntary, rhythmic, oscillating motions of the eyes

36. **Parenchyma**—Functional tissue of an organ, distinguished from connective and supporting tissue

37. **Plateau**—Point in recovery when progress slows or stops; often used as criterion for discontinuing therapy services

38. **Postictal**—Phase that follows an attack such as acute epilepsy; subjective sensation can be variable

39. **Ptosis**—Drooping eyelid

40. **Recanalization**—Restoration of blood flow to an arterial occlusion site

41. **Spasticity**—Unusual tightness, or stiffness, of muscle due to increased tone, or hypertonia; occurs within days to weeks in 30% of stroke patients

42. **Sulcus** (plural is **sulci**)—Deep grooves on the surface of the cerebral hemisphere

43. **Supratentorial**—Refers to portions of the brain above the tentorium (*see* Tentorium)

44. **Symmetry**—Two sides having the same size and shape

45. **Tentorium**—Extension of the dura mater that separates the cerebellum from the inferior portion of the occipital lobes

46. **Thrombolysis**—Dissolution, or lysis, of a blood clot

47. **Tonic**—Pertaining to, or characterized by, tension or contraction, especially muscular tension

48. **Ventricles**—Four hollow spaces in the brain that are filled with cerebrospinal fluid

49. **Vertigo**—Sensation of moving around in space, or having objects move around the person; indicates disturbance of the equilibratory apparatus

50. **White matter**—Bundles of myelinated axons that connect various grey matter areas of the brain and carry nerve impulses between neurons

References

Acker, J., Pancioli, A., Crocco, T. J., Eckstein, M. K., Jauch, E. C., Larrabee, H., . . . Stranne, S. K. (2007). Implementation strategies for emergency medical services within stroke systems of care: A policy statement from the American Heart Association/American Stroke Association expert panel on emergency medical services systems and the stroke council. *Stroke, 38*, 3097–3115.

Adams, H. P., Bendixen, B. H., Kappelle, L. J., Biller, J., Love, B. B., Gordon, D. L., & Marsh, E. E. (1993). Classification of subtype of acute ischemic stroke: Definitions for use in a multicenter clinical trial. *Stroke, 24*, 35–41.

Alberts, M. J., Latchaw, R. E., Jagoda, A., Wechsler, L. R., Crocco, T., George, M. G., . . . Walker, M. D. (2011). Revised and updated recommendations for the establishment of primary stroke centers: A summary statement from the brain attack coalition. *Stroke, 42*, 2651–2665.

Alexander, S. (Ed.). (2013). *Evidence-based nursing care for stroke and neurovascular conditions.* Ames, IA: Wiley-Blackwell.

Alexander, S., Gallek, M., Presciutti, M., & Zrelak, P. (2012). Care of the patient with aneurysmal subarachnoid hemorrhage. *AANN Clinical Practice Guideline Series.* Retrieved from http://www.aann.org/pubs/content/guidelines.html

Bakas, T., Austin, J. K., Okonkwo, K. F., Lewis, R. R., & Chadwick, L. (2002). Needs, concerns, strategies, and advice of stroke caregivers the first 6 months after discharge. *Journal of Neuroscience Nursing, 34,* 242–51.

Barnum, B. (1997). Licensure, certification, and accreditation. *Online Journal of Issues in Nursing, 2*(3). Retrieved from www.nursingworld.org/MainMenuCategories/ANAMarketplace/ANAPeriodicals/OJIN/TableofContents/Vol21997/No3Aug97/LicensureCertificationandAccreditation.aspx

Beaglehole, B. (1988). Modification of Rankin scale: Recovery of motor function after stroke. *Stroke, 19*(12), 1497–1500.

Bolek, B. (2006). Facing cranial nerve assessment. *American Nurse Today, 1*(2), 21–22.

Brain Attack Coalition. (2013). *About the coalition.* Retrieved from www.stroke-site.org

Bushnell, C. D., Olson, D. M., Zhao, X., Pan, W., Zimmer, L. O., Goldstein, L. B., . . . Peterson, E. D. (2011). Secondary preventive medication persistence and adherence 1 year after stroke. *Neurology, 77*(12), 1182–1190.

Butcher, K., Christensen, S., Parsons, M., De Silva, D. A., Ebinger, M., Levi, C., . . . Davis, S. M. (2010). Postthrombolysis blood pressure elevation is associated with hemorrhagic transformation. *Stroke, 41,* 72–77.

Camp, R. (1989). *Benchmarking: The search for industry best practices that leads to superior performance.* Milwaukee, WI: ASQC Quality Press.

Cheung, R., & Liang-Yu, Z. (2003). Use of the original, modified, or new intracerebral hemorrhage score to predict mortality and morbidity after intracerebral hemorrhage. *Stroke, 34,* 1717–1722.

CLOTS Trials Collaboration. (2009). Effectiveness of thigh-length graduated compression stockings to reduce the risk of deep vein thrombosis after stroke (CLOTS trial 1): A multicentre, randomised controlled trial. *Lancet, 373*(9679), 1958–1965.

Connolly, E. S., Rabinstein, A. A., Carhuapoma, J. R., Derdeyn, C. P., Dion, J., Higashida, R. T. . . . Vespa, P. (2012). Guidelines for the management of aneurysmal subarachnoid hemorrhage: A guideline for healthcare professionals from the American Heart Association/American Stroke Association. *Stroke, 43,* 1711–1737.

Davis, S. M., Broderick, J., Hennerici, M., Brun, N. C., Diringer, M. N., Mayer, S. A., . . . Steiner, T. (2006). Hematoma growth is a determinant of mortality and poor outcome after intracerebral hemorrhage. *Neurology, 66*(8), 1175–1181.

Demaerschalk, B., Hwang, H., & Leung, G. (2012). Cost analysis, review of stroke centers, telestroke, and rt-PA. *American Journal of Managed Care, 16*(7), 537–544.

DeMers, G., Meurer, W., Shih, R., Rosenbaum, S., & Vilke, G. (2012). Tissue plasminogen activator and stroke: Review of the literature for the clinician. *Journal of Emergency Medicine, 43*(6), 1149–1154.

Donnell, R. (2009). *Barriers to evidence-based use of thrombolytics in ischemic stroke.* Retrieved from http://doctorrw.blogpost.com/2009/06/barriers-to-evidence-based-use-of.html

Donovan, N., Daniels, S., Edmiaston, J., Weinhardt, J., Summers, D., & Mitchell, P. (2013). Dysphagia screening: State of the art: Invitational Conference Proceeding from the State-of-the-Art Nursing Symposium, International Stroke Conference 2012. *Stroke.* Retrieved from http://stroke.ahajournals.org/content/early/2013/02/14/STR.0b013e3182877f57.citation

Duncan, P. (2007). *Stroke effects on cognition, mood & movement: Implications for practice.* Lecture presentation at Duke University. Retrieved from www.americangeriatrics.org/files/documents/research/pps/duncan.pps

Easton, J. D., Saver, J. L., Albers, G. W., Alberts, M. J., Chaturvedi, S., Feldmann, E., . . . Sacco, R. L. (2009). Definition and evaluation of transient ischemic attack: A scientific statement for healthcare professionals from the American Heart Association/American Stroke Association Stroke Council; Council on Cardiovascular Surgery and Anesthesia; Council on Cardiovascular Radiology and Intervention; Council on Cardiovascular Nursing; and the Interdisciplinary Council on Peripheral Vascular Disease. *Stroke, 40*(6), 2276–2293.

Edlow, J. A., Smith, E. E., Stead, L. G., Gronseth, G., Messe, S. R., Jagoda, A. S., . . . Decker, W. W. (2013). Clinical policy: Use of intravenous tPA for the management of acute ischemic stroke in the emergency department. *Annals of Emergency Medicine, 61*, 225–243.

Edmondson, D., Richardson, S., Fausett, J., Falzon, L., Howard, V., & Kronish, I. (2013). *Prevalence of PTSD in survivors of stroke and transient ischemic attack: A meta-analytic review.* Retrieved from http://www.plosone.org/article/info%3Adoi%2F10.1371%2Fjournal.pone.0066435

Ellrodt, A. G., Fonarow, G. C., Schwamm, L. H., Albert, N., Bhatt, D. L., Cannon, C. P., . . . Smith, E. E. (2013). Synthesizing lessons learned from Get With The Guidelines: The value of disease-based registries in improving quality and outcomes. *Circulation*. Retrieved from http://circ.ahajournals.org/content/early/2013/10/25/01/cir.0000435779.48007.5c.citation

Furie, K. L., Kasner, S. E., Adams, R. J., Albers, G. W., Bush, R. L., Fagan, S. C., . . . Turan, T. N. (2011). Guidelines for the prevention of stroke in patients with stroke or transient ischemic attack: A guideline for healthcare professionals from the American Heart Association/American Stroke Association. *Stroke, 42*, 227–276.

Gage, B. F., Waterman, A. D., Shannon, W., Boechler, M., Rich, M. W., & Radford, M. J. (2001). Validation of clinical classification schemes for predicting stroke: Results from the National Registry of Atrial Fibrillation. *Journal of the American Medical Association, 285*, 2864–2870.

Go, A., Mozaffarian, D., Roger, V., Benjamin, E., Berry, J., Borden, W., . . . Turner, M. (2013). Heart disease and stroke statistics— 2013 update: A report from the American Heart Association. *Circulation, 127*, e132-e152.

Goldstein, L. B., Bushnell, C. D., Adams, R. J., Appel, L. J., Braun, L. T., Chaturvedi, S., . . . Pearson, T. A. (2011). Guidelines for the primary prevention of stroke: A guideline for healthcare professionals from the American Heart Association/American Stroke Association. *Stroke, 42*, 517–584.

Hinchey, J., Shephard, T., Furie, K., Smith, D., Wang, D., & Tong, S. (2005). Formal dysphagia screening protocols prevent pneumonia. *Stroke, 36*(9), 1972–1976.

Jauch, E. C., Saver, J. L., Adams, H. P., Bruno, A., Connors, J. J., Demaerschalk, B. M., . . . Yonas, H. (2013). Guidelines for the early management of patients with acute ischemic stroke: A guideline for healthcare professionals from the American Heart Association/American Stroke Association. *Stroke, 44*, 870–947.

Johnston, S. C., Rothwell, P. M., Nguyen-Huynh, M. N., Giles, M. F., Elkins, J. S., Bernstein, A. L., & Sidney, S. (2007). Validation and refinement of scores to predict very early stroke risk after transient ischaemic attack. *Lancet, 369*, 283–292.

Kidwell, C., Shephard, T., Tonn, S., Lawyer, B., & Murdock, M. (2003). Establishment of primary stroke centers: A survey of physician attitudes and hospital resources. *Neurology, 60*, 1452–1456.

Kruyt, N. D., Nederkoorn, P. J., Dennis, M., Leys, D., Ringleb, P. A., Rudd, A. G., . . . Roos, Y. B. (2013). Door-to-needle time and the proportion of patients receiving intravenous thrombolysis in acute ischemic stroke: Uniform interpretation and reporting. *Stroke, 44*, 3249–3253.

Langhorne, P., Asplund, K., Berman, P., Blomstrand, C., Dennis, M., Douglas, J., . . . Wilhelmsen, L. (1997). Collaborative systematic review of the randomised trials of organised inpatient (stroke unit) care after stroke. *British Medical Journal, 314*, 1151.

Latchaw, R. E., Alberts, M. J., Lev, M. H., Connors, J. J., Harbaugh, R. E., Higashida, R. T., . . . Walters, B. (2009). Recommendations for imaging of acute ischemic stroke: A scientific statement from the American Heart Association. *Stroke, 40*, 3646–3678.

Mahoney, F., & Barthel, D. (1965). Functional evaluation: The Barthel index. *Maryland State Medical Journal, 14*, 56–61.

Miller, E. L., Murray, L., Richards, L., Zorowitz, R. D., Bakas, T., Clark, P., & Billinger, S. A. (2010). Comprehensive overview of nursing and interdisciplinary rehabilitation care of the stroke patient: A scientific statement from the American Heart Association. *Stroke, 41*, 2402–2448.

Morgenstern, L. B., Hemphill, J. C., Anderson, C., Becker, K., Broderick, J. P., Connolly, E. S., . . . Tamargo, R. J. (2010). Guidelines for the management of spontaneous intracerebral hemorrhage: A guideline for healthcare professionals from the American Heart Association/American Stroke Association. *Stroke, 41*, 2108–2219.

National Institute of Neurological Disorders and Stroke. (2013). *NIH Stroke Scale.* Retrieved from http://www.ninds.nih.gov/doctors/NIH_stroke_scale.pdf

National Institutes of Health. (2003). *NHLBI issues new high blood pressure clinical practice guidelines.* Retrieved from http://www.nih.gov/news/pr/may2003/nhlbi-14.htm

Nilsen, M. (2010). A historical account of stroke and the evolution of nursing care for stroke patients. *Journal of Neuroscience Nursing, 42*(1), 19–27.

Ovbiagele, B., Goldstein, L. B., Higashida, R. T., Howard, V. J., Johnston, S. C., Khavjou, O. A., . . . Trogdon, J. G. (2013). Forecasting the future of stroke in the United States: A policy statement from the American Heart Association and American Stroke Association. *Stroke, 44*, 2361–2375.

Philp, I., Brainin, M., Walker, M. F., Ward, A. B., Gillard, P., Shields, A. L., & Norrving, B. (2013). Development of a poststroke checklist to standardize follow-up care for stroke survivors. *Journal of Stroke and Cerebrovascular Disease, 22*(7), e173–e180.

Pugh, S., Mathiesen, C., Meighan, M., Summers, D., & Zrelak, P. (2012). *Guide to the care of the hospitalized patient with ischemic stroke* (2nd ed., rev.). AANN Clinical Practice Guideline Series. Retrieved from http://www.aann.org/pubs/content/guidelines .html

Rankin, J. (1957). Cerebral vascular accidents in patients over the age of 60. *Scottish Medical Journal, 2,* 200–215.

Rosen, D., & MacDonald, R. (2005). Subarachnoid hemorrhage Grading Scales: A systematic review. *Neurocritical Care, 2,* 110–118.

Rosenfeld, C. (Ed.). (2013). *Overview of clinical trials.* Retrieved from http://www.centerwatch.com/clinical-trials/overview.aspx

Sacco, R. L., Kasner, S. E., Broderick, J. P., Caplan, L. R., Connors, J. J., Culebras, A., . . . Vinters, H. V. (2013). An updated definition of stroke for the 21st century: A statement for healthcare professionals from the American Heart Association/American Stroke Association. *Stroke, 44,* 2064–2089.

Schwamm, L. H., Fayad, P., Acker, J. E., Duncan, P., Fonarow, G. C., Girgus, M., . . . Yancy, C. W. (2010). Translating evidence into practice: A decade of efforts by the American Heart Association/American Stroke Association to reduce death and disability due to stroke. *Stroke, 41,* 1051–1065.

Scommegna, P. (2012) *More U.S. children raised by grandparents.* Retrieved from http://www.prb.org/Publications/Articles/2012/US-children-grandparents.aspx

Shiel, W.C., Jr., & Stöppler, M.C. (Eds.) (2008). *Webster's New World Medical Dictionary* (3rd ed.). Hoboken, NJ: Wiley. Retrieved from www.medicinenet.com

Stein, J. (2013). *New therapies in stroke rehabilitation.* Retrieved from http://nyp.org/services/rehabmed/stroke-therapies.html

Xu, P. (2012). Using teach-back for patient education and self-management. *American Nurse Today, 7*(3). Retrieved from http://www .americannursetoday.com/Article.aspx?id=8848&fid=8812

Index